Reiki Healing For Beginners:

Heal yourself and the others, increase your energy, improve your health, reduce stress and unlock the secret about physical, mental, emotional and spiritual therapy.

By reading this document, the reader agrees that under no circumstances is the author responsible for any losses, direct or indirect, which are incurred as a result of the use of information contained within this document, including, but not limited to, —errors, omissions, or inaccuracies.

Introduction

Congratulations on purchasing " Reiki Healing for Beginners: Heal yourself and the others, increase your energy, improve your health, reduce stress and unlock the secret about physical, mental, emotional and spiritual therapy." and thank you for doing so.

Individuals use Reiki for unwinding, stress decrease, and manifestation alleviation, in endeavors to improve generally speaking wellbeing and prosperity. Individuals have utilized Reiki with nervousness, interminable agony, HIV/AIDS, and other wellbeing conditions, just as by individuals recuperating from a medical procedure or encountering reactions from malignancy medicines. Reiki has likewise been given to individuals who are biting the dust, as well as to their families and guardians, to help give a feeling of harmony.

The person being healed, wherein we will refer to as Customers, may encounter a secret government of unwinding during a Reiki session. They may likewise feel warm, tingly, lethargic, or revived. Reiki gives off an impression of being commonly protected, and no genuine symptoms have been accounted for.

No unique foundation or accreditations are expected to get preparing. Be that as it may, Reiki must be gained from an accomplished instructor or a Master; it can't act naturally educated. The particular strategies educated can shift significantly. Preparing in conventional Reiki has three degrees or levels, each concentrating on an alternate part of the training. Every degree incorporates at least one inception. Additionally, these are called attunements or strengthening influences. Getting inception is accepted to enact the capacity to get to Reiki vitality.

There are a lot of books regarding this matter available, thanks again for picking this one! Each exertion was made to guarantee it is loaded with however much helpful data as could be expected!

Chapter 1: Getting Started: Your Ultimate Guide to Reiki

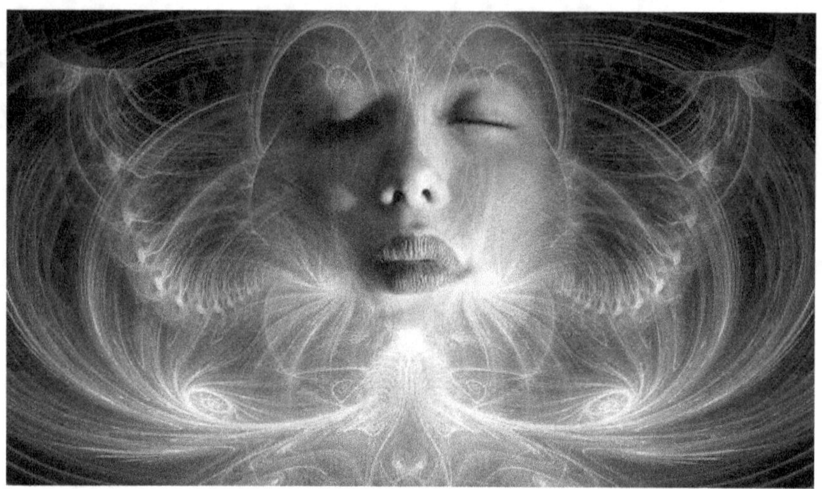

What is Reiki?

Reiki is a gentle form of therapy that involves touch and is meant to assist the body to heal itself from common ailments that it is dealing with. Reiki practitioners are able to tap into the natural energy of the body in order to remove any blockage that may be there and to redirect the flow of misdirected or stagnant energy that is there. This can help to promote the health and wellness inside the individual. Reiki is going to rely on helping the chakras, or the energy centers, of the body. These energy centers are going to allow the practitioner to stimulate the healing abilities that are found naturally inside of the body. Through straightening, healing, and clearing the flow of energy through the body, it is possible to resolve many of the common ailments that are going on inside of the body, including emotional, mental, and physical problems.

When you do not take care of your energy imbalances, it is going to cause some physical ailments inside of the body. In fact, many of the diseases and illnesses that go on inside the body are due to these energy imbalances. Reiki is able to come in and solve some of these problems, opening up those energy centers so that you feel much better. Reiki is also known as a form of mental therapy because it has the ability to impact your psychological conditions, like depression and anxiety, in a positive manner. In fact, those who have practiced Reiki often feel a better sense of well-being and improved self-confidence when they are done.

Reiki can work well for so many people because it is gentle and non-invasive, which is completely different compared to the other forms of alternative healing Rather than focusing all that energy on the symptoms of a condition, Reiki is going to treat the whole person, helping to send healing energy in the direction that it is needed the most.

Preparation Before Your Session

To first prepare your mind, you'll want to speak the Reiki Ideals. Say the words from your heart and mind, as well as your lips. As you are repeating the Reiki Ideas, put your hands, palms together, in front of your heart chakra as illustrated on the following pages. Before you begin, invite your inner spirit to participate in this self-healing process. You will be the healer and the healed as you practice Reiki's self-healing discipline.

Think of this as a Reiki prayer. It should be done with a reverent and open heart. This is not a time to be skeptical or doubtful, but rather a time of knowing that you are about to be introduced to your helper and comforter, your strength and guide. Breathe deeply; focus on slowly inhaling through your nose and then just as slowly exhaling through your mouth. When you have released all the air from your lungs, let your breath drift off then hold it for about five to six seconds longer before slowly releasing the remaining air from your passageways.

Invite Reiki to guide your energy throughout every cell of your body, touching the areas that require healing. Continue to feel the relaxing rhythm of your heart as Reiki responds to your gentle requests for calmness, peace, and healing.

To be completely prepared for your session, do this first Reiki pose each evening for three or four days before your full session to come. This will help to open your chakras and encourage your mind to freely and fearlessly seek Reiki before your first session and be fully prepared to release what binds you.

Only ask and invite during these first few evenings, staying calm and relaxed, prayerfully seeking Reiki's wisdom and healing power for your first full session. Remember to thank Reiki for all that you are about to experience. Make sure you get plenty of rest and drink lots of water to wash away the negatives.

Symbols: Reiki has its own three sets of symbols representing its own arena or its own category of assumptions. The first is Tattwa. Tattwa has five different symbols each representing a different element of the universe. They represent earth, air, water, fire, spirit. They reign over the realm of energy in the brain. This group of symbols may also affect other areas such as realities that are not physical like dreams.

The next symbol group is physical items such as Rosaries. They have the ability to be charged with the power to cause an effect. The final group of devices like the Reiki symbols learned earlier, that can enable the use of Reiki energy. These symbols offer a pathway to connection with energy that is independent.

The symbols are not the exclusive means of accessing Reiki energy. They will make your Reiki experience much more gratifying or satisfying. If you don't know the exact meaning of any given symbol you may still use it; you will gain wisdom with time and practice.

The Master Symbol of Reiki holds the greatest power. It is used for a much deeper, spiritual healing. It enhances one's intuition and can change your life dramatically. The Master Reiki symbol is made of three kanji's (characters). One means great or greatly. The second means light in noun form or smooth as an adjective. This kanji may also mean completely. The final kanji is an adjective or a verb. It may mean evident or see, understand. Put together, the three kanji' s mean great bright light.

Remember, you may use all or only selected symbols, they are not a necessary ingredient in Reiki. They do bring enhancement to the energy flow. You may, of course, choose to use none.

Like earlier mentioned symbols, these can be activated in numerous ways. You might draw or visualize a symbol, or you may chant. You might form the shape in your mouth with the tip of your tongue. How you activate is up to you.

Prepare your chakras: Prior to using Reiki meditation on yourself, you are going to want to ensure that your chakras are open and ready for the experience as well. The following technique will also work well with the Kundalini meditation discussed in the next chapter. While you are welcome to work through the entire process each time, you may instead simply want to focus on the parts that deal with the chakras that are bothering you the most.

For starters, you will work on the root chakra which you can start doing by simply focusing on the color red. When you start focusing on the color the odds are pretty good that it is a dull, dark red as opposed to a strong, vibrant red which should be your ultimate goal. Throughout your time working with this chakra you are going to want to focus on the color until it is bright and pulsating.

After you have opened up your root chakra, you will be ready to move on to the sacral chakra which is associated with the color orange which you will want to focus on making shine as brightly as possible. In fact, each chakra has its own color and you will want to focus on it as you work to make that particular chakra shine. You will want to make your way up the body until you reach the crown chakra. Once you have done so you can expect all of your chakras to be fully opened which means you are ready to move forward with Reiki meditation.

It is important to understand that this method is not something that you are going to see results with overnight. Depending on how tarnished your chakras are it could take weeks of diligent effort to get them shining brightly. Thus, if this is your first time with this practice or you simply haven' t done it in a while then it is important to leave yourself enough time to do it properly without feeling rushed.

Gassho meditation: Another technique that you are able to use is known as Gassho Meditation. This method is going to take about five to fifteen minutes where you will focus all of your attention just on Reiki. It is beneficial to do this for each day, although there are programs that will help you to get started and they recommend doing it for 21-days to see how you like it.

The steps to Gassho meditation are pretty simple. You do not need to do a ton of things other than concentrate on the Reiki healing powers, do some deep breathing, and sit in the right position. The steps that you need for Gassho Meditation include:

•	Take your hands and hold them in a prayer position. This is traditionally leaving the hands, with palms together, touching and the fingers touching as well. Make sure that these prayer hands are right at the heart.
•	When the hands are done, close your eyes.
•	Start to breathe in the Reiki energy through your nose, taking in a nice deep breath rather than the fast and uneven breaths that you have been doing before.
•	Once you are ready, it is time to exhale that breath

through your whole body. This would include the physical body, the etheric body, the mental body, and the spiritual body.

You would just keep on with the deep breathing for as long as you needed, concentrating on the Reiki healing power as you go. Of course, there are a few different variations that you can try with this. Some people like to add these in because they allow them something to concentrate on or because they think that it adds some more power.

You can choose to write down a goal and then ask that some sort of clarification comes to you throughout your session. You can add in some music, as long as it is soft and inspiring in some manner or even chants a mantra. If you are dealing with a big problem in your life, you could ask for some help and guidance to get through that problem. And some people decide to draw the power symbol, the mental or emotional symbol, or the distance symbol over their body when they first get started. You are able to choose the variation that works the best for you, or you can stick with the steps that are listed above to help you.

Reiki Meditation Example

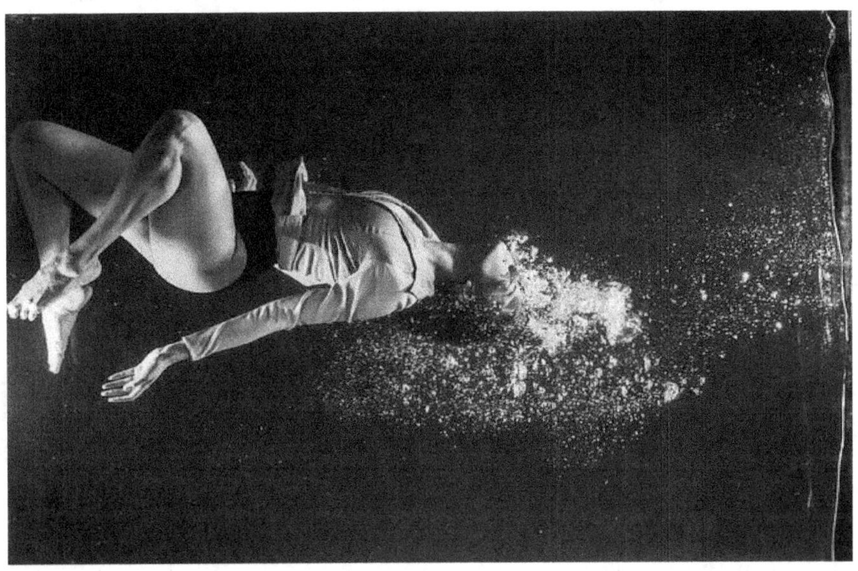

Lay or sit down comfortably on a mat. Keep your back straight. Stay relaxed, composed, and calm. Breathe deeply. Imagine that you are inhaling the goodness and happiness that you want. Now exhale all the negative emotions like anxiety, fear, and depression. Imagine them leaving your body. Do this a few times and think about how in tune your mind and body are. Just relax.

There are seven different chakras in the body. They go from the bottom of your spine to the top of your head. These are energy centers for the body. Put your hand in front of each chakra and hold it for a few minutes. This all depends on what your body needs. If your body asks for it to stay longer, leave it there. Move it if the body has enough. Feeling with the hands is the best way to listen and connect to your body. As you tune in with your hands, imagine the universe's life force is entering your body through the hands.

Your chakras are the passageway. Feel your body vibrate with the energy flow. Go into deep relaxation and rejuvenation.

Put your palms together at the top of your head. Hold your hands there and listen to your body. Pay attention. Continue to do this and breathe slowly and deeply. Remove all the negative and bring all the positives into you. Relax.
Put your hands on your forehead. Now move them to the back of your head. Move down to the throat and put on hand on the throat and the other at the back of the neck. Hold this for a time and relax.

Continue down and put your hands on the back of your shoulders. Your fingers should be facing downward. Your touch needs to be gentle. Hold your hands still until the body is ready for it to be moved.

Put your hands on your chest covering your heart. Remember to hold until the body tells you to move.

Move on to the rib area, then the stomach and lower abdomen. Keeping your touch gentle and moving when the body is ready.

When you are done with the head and torso, move to the hips and put your hands on both your hips. Moving only when the body tells you to. Feel the energy flowing through the body. Enjoy the sensations.

Move on to your knees and feet. For your feet, place the hands either on bottom or top whichever is more comfortable. Move your hands when your body is ready. Enjoy the experience.

Finally, place your hands in the prayer position and put them in front of your chest. Sit with the spine straight and the body taut. Breathe normally. Feel the energy coursing through your body. Continue this for another three to five minutes or as long as you feel the need. This process is done when you feel energized and ignited.

Chapter 2: The Three Degrees

The father of modern Reiki, Mikao Usui, was born on August 15th, 1865, in what is known today as the town of Taniai-Mura located in the Yamagata area of Gifu in the modern-day prefecture of Kyoto. Not much is known about Mikao Usui, but it is believed that he was born within a wealthy family as only the male children of wealthy families were able to have access to above average education.

From an early age, Usui trained within the Buddhist religion at the Tendai Buddhist school. He began schooling within this discipline as a very young child. He quickly began training in disciplined of ever-increasing difficulty. He is recalled as a gifted child who showed promise in a number of areas such as prescription, fortune telling, studies of the brain and the mind, and deep religious philosophy. As a result of his studies, he was able to take advantage of every opportunity to learn the ways of the world and the way the human body and mind functioned together. His understanding of the Buddhist Bible, the Kyoten, was very deep and insightful. He eventually married to a young lady named Sadako. The couple had a girl born around 1907.

As an adult, Usui had deep curiosity about the ways of the world outside of his home country. He ventured out into China and some western countries. In doing so, he was able to learn about the ways in which people conducted themselves in cultures different to his. Usui held a number of different positions such as office worker, neighborhood officer, a reporter, secretary to a legislator, chairman to convicts and even an industrialist. He would serve as secretary to Shimpei Goto, who was a renowned government official in the position of Secretary of the Railroad, then later serving the Postmaster General and ultimately becoming Secretary of the Interior and the State.

Nevertheless, Usui ended up foregoing this lifestyle and took up the habits of the Buddhist Monks. He would eventually enter the Buddhist priesthood thus cementing his life' s purpose. He would consistently reflect on the meaning of life while undergoing the 21 days of suffering. It is said that during these sufferings, Usui received a divine inspiration for a plan of physical recovery which would eventually be known as " Reiki" . This story is said to have happened on Mount Kurama during one of his sufferings.

The overall inspiration is believed to have been a combination of a series of traditional oriental treatments, fused into one, and harmonized to create a holistic approach to healing the body. As such, Reiki shares its origins with traditional Chinese medicine, the oriental discipline Chi Gong and the Japanese Kiko needle treatment. By experimenting with the techniques of all these disciplines, Usui discovered the extraordinary results on a number of ailments.

By April 1922, Usui began teaching this healing art at the first school of its kind in Harajuku, Tokyo. At first, Usui had a small handbook which was later translated into English and disseminated in the Western world. The handbook's original title was " The Original Reiki Handbook of Dr. Mikao Usui" as published by the early Reiki master Frank Arjava Petter, who was living in Japan at the time.

Due to Usui's track record of success, his fame as a doctor and healer began spreading across Japan. Given the fact that Japan was undergoing a deep and profound social change, this apparent revolution coincided with Japan's aperture to the West.
Reiki thus began gaining a foothold among people of all sorts, but in particular, Reiki quickly gained momentum with

older individuals who believed in preserving their ties to ancient healing practices.

At the first Reiki school, learners were taught Reiki as a means of healing, but also as a way of preserving Japan's cultural legacy and history. History records that this school gained notoriety as the number of learners that attended it began to increase.

In September of 1923, a massive earthquake rocked Tokyo and Yokohoma. It is believed that this earthquake measure 7.9 on the Richter Scale. It left thousands of dead and even more wounded. It is believed that the number of casualties from this earthquake was around 140,000. At its time, it was the single-most destructive event in Japanese history. But it also afforded Usui, and his students, the opportunity to put their Reiki discipline to the test. They would go out to treat those who had been injured in the earthquake. As a result of this effort, Reiki began to garner a great deal of attention.

By 1925, Usui's following had grown to the degree that he was looking to open a second school in Nakano, located outside of Tokyo. As Usui began to spend time away from the first school, his senior students began taking over his duties.

These senior students began training other novice learners in the ways of Reiki. However, Usui passed away before he could complete the opening of the second school. His death in 1926 spurred the construction of a monument in his honor near his grave at the Saihoji Temple y Suginamiku, Tokyo. His followers would honor Usui' s legacy by continuing to teach Reiki.

Reiki would eventually be divided into 6 different levels of mastery. The first four are known as " Shoden" with the last two are known as " Okuden" in addition to the Shinpi-nook. In the beginning levels, disciplines are asked to master their presence and relationship with the material (Shoden) before progressing into the deeper, inward levels (Okuden). After these levels, the disciple arrives at the Shinpi-lair level, or the mystery level. Under this construction, around 2,000 individuals were trained in the ways of Reiki with a total of about 15 to 17 Reiki masters. Although, it should be noted that there was no such title of " Reiki Master" at the time in Japan.

Reiki is known to be a difficult discipline to master. There are three tiers before students arrive at mastery of Reiki. Nevertheless, time and effort are needed before arriving at full mastery of each level. Here is a description of the three tiers or degrees.

The first degree, known as Reiki, I or Shoden is the introductory phrase in which students learn about history and the underlying philosophy of Reiki. Also, students are taught how to offer Reiki to others and channel the healing energy to the ailing individual.

The second degree, known as Reiki II, or Okuden, students are introduced to the " secret" ways of Reiki. The student is then asked to deepen their learning of the healing energy offered through Reiki. At the completion of this degree, the student is regarded as a " Reiki Master" .

The third degree, known as Reiki III, or Shinpinden, is when the master attains the level needed to become a teacher of Reiki. In this degree, training is often split up into parts, one is the attunement of the healing energy while the second part is devoted to honing the master' s teaching ability.

Now, let' s take a deeper look into the each of the Reiki degrees.

First Degree Of Reiki: Shoden Self Treatment

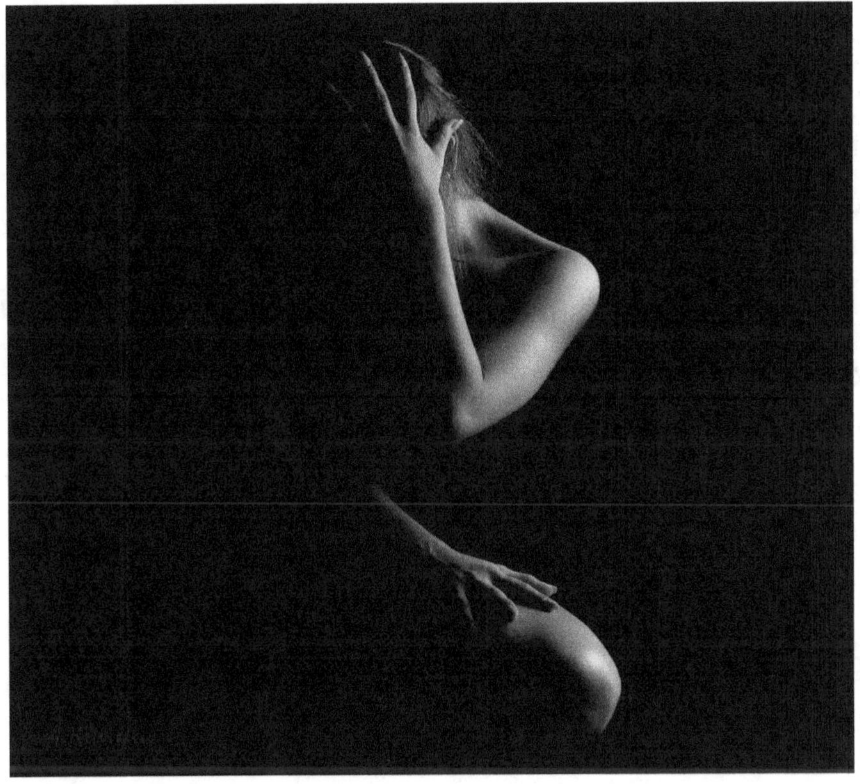

Shoden is a Japanese word signifying " first lessons " .
 It is the main degree of lessons in the customary Japanese
part of Reiki called Usui Reiki Ryoho.

Vitality is a word that not many individuals can clarify in the
entirety of its complexities. You could peruse a book on it or
be informed all concerning it however it is simply the

genuine encounter that educates you.

In this way, a total treatment is given and gotten by each taking an interest understudy and numerous hands-on activities are utilized in a gathering situation during Shoden. This useful experience prompts an internal comprehension of vitality.

A great part of the course is spent working from this perspective, instructing you to work instinctively and to bring that instinctual balance into your regular day-to-day existence. For a fact, it takes, in any event, two days to pick up this degree of certainty. The strategies used to encourage this depend on both the experiential information, which you gain all through the course just as your very own understanding of specialized capacity.

Conventional Japanese Reiki reflection strategies are educated and rehearsed over the two days to expand on this lively information and to help your mending procedure.

In the wake of finishing Shoden in-person, the understudy is approached to keep rehearsing on oneself and complete the online lessons at the Ki Campus. This proceeds with the lively clearing, which was started during the course itself.

Mending resembles 'making entire'; making a balance in your life. The International House of Reiki sees the contemplating of the arrangement of Reiki as an otherworldly venture –   one that is embraced by you with each help offered during, and after, the course by the educators.

Advantages of Shoden Reiki:

Figure out how to unwind.
Increase an unmistakable comprehension of vitality work.
Experience enthusiastic and physical discharge.
Feel good with yourself.
Build up your caring and cherishing perspectives.
Help other people.
Feel solid.
Be educated about the arrangement of Reiki.
Get individual continuous consideration and direction from your instructor.

Have a place with a universal mending network, the International House of Reiki, and get every one of the advantages of the middle's incredible emotionally supportive networks. Shoden understudies are urged to resist for a base charge for proceeding with instruction purposes.

Second Degree of Reiki: Okuden Self Treatment

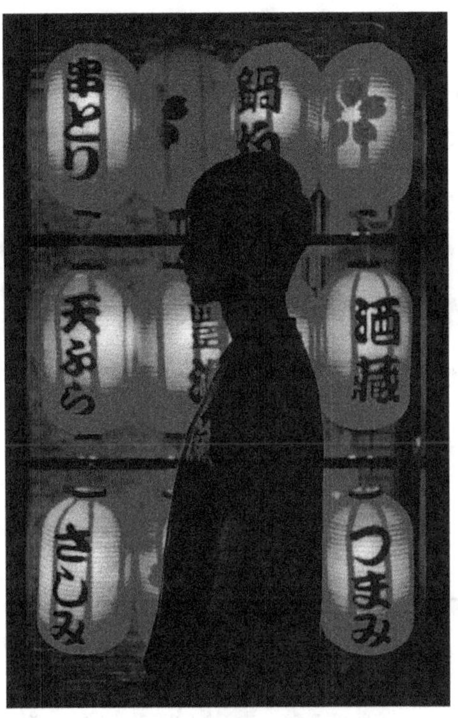

The Second Degree (Okuden) Reiki; instructs understudies to grasp instinctive working, increasing trust in removed, non-contact Reiki with the utilization of hallowed vitality images to reinforce your association and help you on your adventure. This is anything but essential expertise for the vast majority to have, and it is more inside and out than the clear First-Degree Reiki.

Experiencing Okuden preparing is prescribed for understudies who have taken Shoden level 1 course and have been rehearsing day by day self-treatment for at least a half year. The Reiki Intuitive recommends understudies who have prepared with another Master to either have a discussion or go to her Reiki Share bunch before focusing on the preparation in full.

Okuden is a Japanese word signifying 'inward lessons'. As the word suggests a more profound comprehension and association with Usui Mikao's lessons is accomplished during this course.

This level instructs how to associate with Earth and Heaven vitality, the initial steps to winding up completely incorporated with the universe. This is accomplished through the act of Shirushi (images) and Jumon (mantras). It will empower the understudy to upgrade his/her very own vitality levels and affectability. There are numerous viewpoints to the Shirushi and Jumon which incorporate reciting and perception strategies. As opposed to being outside apparatuses – the attention here is on inner use for otherworldly improvement.

The idea of Oneness, understanding that we are One vigorously with everything known to mankind, is one of the significant advantages of working as such and is normally drilled in the course. A component of this investigation of Oneness enables the professional to see the more profound implications of far off mending. Extra Japanese Reiki strategies are offered to help profound development significantly further.

As mindfulness develops so does the capacity to help other people – this is talked about at this level. In the wake of finishing Okuden, the understudy is required to proceed with the rehearsing on oneself as well as other people where conceivable.

Advantages of Okuden Reiki:

Discover balance in regular daily existence.
Experience the vibe of being grounded in any circumstance.
Start to discharge your dread and outrage.
Comprehend your association with individuals, places, nature, and occasions in your general surroundings.
Progress further along your otherworldly way.

Start to help other people expertly.

Extend your insight into the arrangement of Reiki from a Japanese viewpoint.

Get individual continuous consideration and direction from your educator.

Have a place with a worldwide recuperating network, the International House of Reiki, and get every one of the advantages of the middle's incredible emotionally supportive networks. Okuden understudies are urged to resist for a base charge for proceeding with training purposes.

Third Degree Of Reiki: Shinpiden Self Treatment

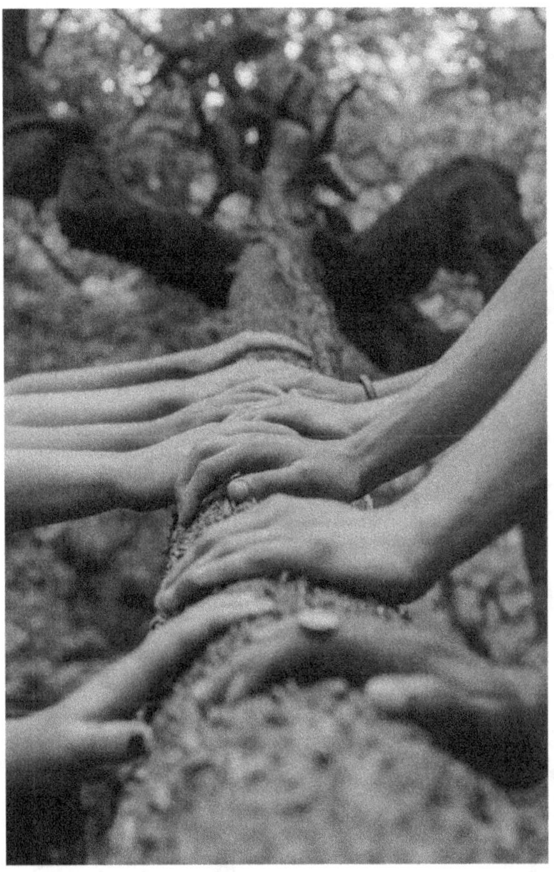

Shinpiden centers on self-awareness and shows the understudy how to perform attunements. At this level, you move into finding increasingly about the puzzles of life. How you identify with yourself and the universe. This can be rehearsed for an amazing remainder and is constantly an individual practice, which can form into an expert showing practice on the off chance that you do want.

There are likewise more profound Japanese social and philosophical understandings that are instructed at each level, which will be clarified in more subtleties with the proper levels.

Shinpiden is the Japanese word for 'riddle lessons'. It is gone for Level II professionals or set up Reiki Masters who wish to proceed with their own voyage, an adventure that is progressing long after you complete the Shinpiden course. It is thusly not just about educating and is even appropriate for the individuals who wish to just build up their own Reiki practice and once in a while instruct people around them.

Self-strengthening is accomplished in Shinpiden through a solid enthusiastic association with the wellspring of Reiki. It is additionally the consequence of the certainty you will feel because of your careful learning of Reiki – how it functions, what every one of the minor departures from Reiki really are, the place Reiki remains on the planet today, the Japanese Shirusi (images) and Jumon (mantras) and their association with Japanese methods of reasoning and what the root of Reiki's otherworldly nature is.

One of the major focal points of this course is to take advantage of the feeling that you are, and consistently were, an incredible, brilliant light – this is accomplished by working with the fourth shirushi and jumon.

Advantages of Shinpiden Reiki:

Access a profound feeling of quietness.
Be sure as an instructor and professional.
Start to help other people expertly by instructing just as treating.
Get individual continuous consideration and direction from your instructor.
Have a place with a worldwide mending network, the International House of Reiki, and get every one of the advantages of the middle's incredible emotionally supportive networks.

Chapter 3: Getting to Know The Reiki Master

What Is A Reiki Master?

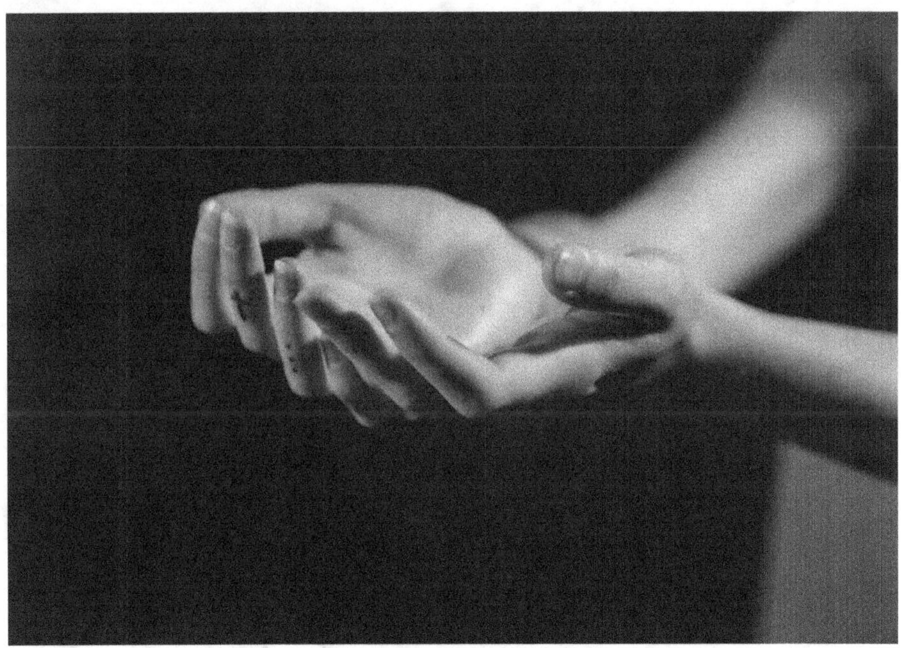

Given the idea of the ace level and the energies that become accessible to us, being a Reiki ace can be a progressing procedure including consistent self-improvement. With the ace attunement and the utilization of the ace image, we get the chance to open increasingly more totally to the boundless capability of this art and to create within each of us the characteristics that are held within the vitality of Reiki. Consider every one of the parts of Reiki vitality - other than the possibility to mend for all intents and purposes all disease, it likewise contains boundless love, delight, harmony, empathy, astuteness, bounty and significantly more. We know these are the characteristics of Reiki on the grounds that individuals experience them when giving or accepting Reiki medications. They are particularly evident when we think about the wellspring of Reiki. When doing as such, many are lifted up into a protected spot where they feel totally thought about and become mindful of the superb potential outcomes that can emerge out of inside.

When we mull over these things it is anything but difficult to move toward becoming overpowered with good faith and the certain comprehension of the fact that any, and all, difficulties of the world can be overcome and that our existence could be a great encounter. The Japanese term of the highest degree in Reiki is Shinpiden that signifies "Puzzle Teaching." The riddle that is talked about is the secret of God's adoration, shrewdness, and power.

It is a riddle since God has no limits; every one of the qualities of God including marvel, excellence, and elegance reach out a long way past our capacity to understand. Regardless of how created in this life or in any future degree of presence, we will never completely get it. This is the reason it is and will consistently stay a superb secret.

When we get the Usui ace image and the attunement that engages it, it makes the likelihood for us to end up mindful of the Ultimate Reality. This is communicated in the meaning of the Usui ace image that demonstrates that it speaks to that piece of the self that is as of now totally illuminated! When we utilize the ace image, we are really interfacing with our own edified selves. This truth be told, is the genuine wellspring of Reiki vitality - it really originates from the most profound and most significant piece of our own inclination, our very own illuminated self. Even though we might be under the impression that this phenomenon is originating from afar and descends to use through the crown chakra, the fact of the matter is that it is merely a hallucination and just shows up along these lines in light of our restricted mindfulness.

The healing energy that is summoned in Reiki is bestowed

upon by the creator. It is therefore this energy that leads us to heal and opens us up to greater self-understanding and enlightenment. However, improvement doesn't happen naturally. Reiki regards our through and through freedom and doesn't compel advancement on us, yet on the off chance that we look for it and expect it, and use Reiki for this reason, at that point absolutely, we will be guided into a more prominent recuperating background. Attempt this analysis. Begin by conducting Reiki on your own self utilizing our ace image in the hands within a position which is agreeable. (On the off chance that you aren' t an ace at Reiki but rather at the first or second level, attempt it in any case without the ace image.) Then ruminate over this insistence. "I give up totally to the Reiki vitality and the source from which it comes." Repeat this assertion again and again, at that point as the Reiki vitality keeps on streaming, with your inward eye, search for the wellspring of Reiki, either inside yourself or above.

By doing this, you will have numerous significant encounters. These are probably going to incorporate ending up progressively mindful of the way Reiki functions inside you and sensing that its astonishing characteristics. New conceivable outcomes for self-awareness will be exhibited and you will be welcome to partake in life in a progressively important manner. As your mindfulness draws much nearer to the actual source, you will wind up mindful of stunning bits of knowledge and have regularly expanding encounters of happiness, security, and harmony. This is a superb exercise and definitely justified even despite the time. We recommend you do this regularly and as you do as such, these encounters will end up more grounded. At that point, on the off chance that you acknowledge the mending changes that are displayed, profound recuperating will start occurring and you will likewise start accepting direction about how to improve your life. While this contemplation is basic, it is additionally exceptionally ground-breaking and can lead you into a cheerful and sound perspective, making enduring changes that will shape the establishment of an increasingly advantageous life.

Reiki can manage you in approaches to make its recuperating power progressively advantageous and to mend all the more profoundly. What's more, simultaneously, one can assume that this discipline will direct you to additional mending strategies which are actually directly available for your use notwithstanding Reiki. You may likewise get direction about changes you have to make that expect you to make a move. Your capacity to settle on choices can improve, making it extremely simple to choose precisely what you need, who to connect with, where to work, and so on and this could bring about a totally new course for your life!

When you are engaged with the recuperating procedure, a great method to decide your advancement is to utilize your external world as a sign of your internal improvement. This works since we show our whole experience through our contemplations and goals - both cognizant and oblivious. When we experience something in our lives, it is on the grounds that some piece of our being has made it. When we acknowledge this thought and assume total liability for what happens in our lives, we enter an extremely amazing spot. We would then be able to get rid of the things which do not provide any benefit and make every part of our lives better.

In the event that your external world contains positive encounters, and you are making a mind-blowing most, this implies your internal world is in a comparative state. The turn around is likewise valid, thereby when we go through agonizing experiences and circumstances, or are disillusioned or experience by situations that cultivate dread, stress or uncertainty, this is additionally in light of the fact that some piece of our inward being is out of parity and necessities recuperating. On the off chance that something upsetting, or undesirable happens in your life, instead of accusing other individuals or conditions outside yourself, direct your consideration internally and search for the piece of yourself that has made this terrible occasion. At that point utilize your Reiki mending abilities to support and recuperate this part. When you do this, the disagreeable encounters will stop and be supplanted by sound positive encounters.

As we proceed on our recuperating way, we will end up mindful of a degree of cognizance that lives profoundly inside every one of us that can bring a great better approach for living. It makes another disposition that is totally positive and carries with it the capacity to take care of numerous issues and make positive outcomes that beforehand we didn't think conceivable.

What Are the Roles Of A Reiki Master?

There are numerous individuals looking for recuperating who wonder, what do Reiki Masters do, what is the job of a Reiki Master healer and what would they be able to assist me with?

These are on the whole extremely significant inquiries to pose. For customers of Reiki, yet in addition for Reiki Masters themselves. Numerous recently prepared Reiki Master healers, and even many experienced experts and educators, don't have a reasonable comprehension about their job as a healer.

Understanding the job a Reiki Master plays in taking an interest in your mending is significant for everybody included. Understanding what a Reiki Master does and doesn't do impacts a mending session and otherworldly and self-awareness. For the customer, however for the Reiki Master healer as well.

So, what does a Reiki Master do precisely? It might shock you, yet a Reiki Master isn't required to fix your medical issues! From my own encounters working with customers all through the world, I have seen that numerous individuals don't completely comprehend the job a Reiki Master healer plays with regards to mending. There is a constant flow of customers who go to a Reiki Master with a rundown of desires.

Reiki Master healers just associate you with The Source. Regardless of whom your Reiki Master healer is, their job is to associate your body, being and vitality with the vitality of The Source. From here, it is up to The Source what gets mended in you and what doesn't. The aftereffects of a Reiki treatment are not the duty of the healer. Some portion of the duty rests with the customer and the rest with The Source. So how open the customer is to being mended, the amount they have confidence in the capacity to recuperate, and that they are so associated with God, The Source, are a portion of the numerous elements that decide the achievement of a mending session. It is the job of your Reiki Master to associate your vitality with the vitality of The Source. From that point, a customers mending is about their more profound association with The Source.

The principal obligation is to oneself, to sustain and create from inside, and to discharge any cynicism from inside.

Regularly in this day and age, we run over a clash that we can decide to either accept or smoothly resolve. We may get malady that we are to mend from comprehensively. We are tested with negative passionate responses that we should relinquish. We are tested with remaining negative feelings from quite a while ago, sentiments; for example, stress, outrage, low self-esteem, we are not to enable these emotions to rot and develop however to release them and recuperate. Most importantly, we need to deal with ourselves, living by the Reiki Principles as given by Mikao Usui, the originator of Reiki, and permitting ourselves Reiki mending each day. All things considered; we are not very useful to any other individual in the event that we are ourselves a wreck! I find that for myself and for other Reiki Masters, this first duty is the hardest to complete. It is a continuous exertion that gets simpler with long stretches of training. The key is to prop up back to the lessons of Usui with a receptive outlook and humble soul.

The subsequent obligation is to individuals who come to us for Reiki. There are individuals from the open who want treatment and understudies who seek commencement and educating.

When somebody seeks a treatment with Reiki, my instructing was to disclose to the customer that Reiki is a comprehensive vitality, going to where it is most required, and to urge the customer to comprehensively deal with their wellbeing. Reiki works uniquely in contrast to allopathic prescription. While allopathic drug fixes the side effect, Reiki mending is aimed at the entire individual. For example, if a customer came griping of knee torment, it might be that the knee is focused on in light of the fact that the hip is twisted. The hip may have turned into that path so as to make up for a shoulder being twisted. This may have occurred because of worry in the individual's life. On the off chance that this pressure is as yet progressing, the Reiki is probably going to mend the pressure first. This bodes well, as leaving the worry there may prompt further bear hip-knee misalignment and further knee harm! Some portion of the duty of the Reiki Master is to make the customer mindful of this all-encompassing procedure and the requirement for a few sessions. This allows the Reiki to recuperate the side effects just as the hidden causes.

At the point when an understudy seeks commencement and educating, this is the start of a profound, passionate, mental and physical adventure. The Reiki Master needs to consider the street went before this point and above all, bolster the understudy on their energizing new venture with Reiki.

A significant number of us have come into Reiki from a foundation of physical or passionate agony. For a few, there was a profound void to fill. A decent Reiki Master will be delicate to the necessities of their understudies. This implies staying away from natural aggravations in the class to think about understudies with compound sensitivities. It means relinquishing injurious comments given by furious spirits. It means being firm yet delicate with understudies from a sincerely despondent life. Most importantly, in the class, the Reiki Master ought to guarantee the understudy feels needed, regarded, acknowledged and adored. After the commencement and educating, the Reiki Master can bolster their understudy by making accessible and focusing on the requirement for ordinary contact and supervision. The rest is up to the understudy and what feels directly for their advancement with Reiki.

The third obligation is towards friends and family and every single other animal; to put it plainly, our condition. Our mending incorporates thinking about this condition. This doesn't mean enabling an injurious relative to manhandle us or adding to social wrongs since every other person appears to! It means being capable, cherishing genuinely, and enabling recuperating to stream any place it is required and with the consent of the healer. For example, a Reiki Master can begin every day by asking that they are a channel, or course, for Reiki vitality and enabling it to stream any place they stroll in nature. A Reiki Master can buy earth amicable items. A Reiki Master can be accessible for relatives for recuperating as feels fitting and be a power for good. A Reiki Master living by the Reiki Principles will win their living truly, respect their educators and older folks, and be charitable to each living thing.

One of the most normally looked for after administrations I offer to customers is relationship mending. Regardless of who the individual and what kind of life they live, everybody has associations with individuals. Regardless of whether with an accomplice, a companion, a relative or a business associate, a huge piece of life comes down to the connections we have with others. So, relationship recuperating is a prevalent region that individuals frequently need assistance with. Anyway, numerous individuals expect a Reiki Master to do something amazing and power two individuals together in 'amicability'. This is a remarkable inverse of concordance. Indeed, utilizing vitality to constrain two individuals together is more much the same as dark enchantment than mending. No Reiki Master should utilize vitality diverting to control the Will of someone else. Regardless of what the goal might be. There are significant explanations behind why individuals meet up. There are similarly significant purposes behind why individuals part. Inside this uniting and separating of connections are numerous significant open doors for self-advancement and otherworldly development.

So, the job of a Reiki Master isn't to conflict with the regular progression of the Universe. The job of a Reiki Master is to help the individuals in a relationship to make harmony with their connections, to comprehend the message, if conceivable, and to enable them to mend and proceed onward if that is the regular course that relationship should take. The best job a Reiki Master could accept that is turning into a channel and manual for assistance individuals comprehend the more profound importance of their connections.

The specialty of Reiki and profound recuperating plans to

enable the individual to rehearse it. By figuring out how your condition communicates with you, and how you cooperate with your condition, you can start to utilize your musings, goal, feeling, and vitality as instruments of progress. Now and again, numerous customers have an ordinary Reiki Master healer who mends them, yet they don't wish to learn Reiki themselves. We have a couple of customers who feel this way. Anyway, there are various hindrances to this that customers ought to know about.

The job of a Reiki Master is to recuperate, enable and improve their customers. In the event that a co-dependent relationship creates among healed and healer, this can be counter-productive for the development and advancement of the customer. By not figuring out how you make vitality at each minute, how you channel it into your life, and how your life turns into an impression of that vitality you channel, you will never arrive at the purpose of being responsible for your heading throughout everyday life. Acknowledge how vitality streams and you can accomplish self-dominance. There is little reason in a Reiki Master healer expelling a negative vitality hinders from inside you if your considerations, expectations, and activities are more than once re-making those equivalent blockages. When you figure out how you make these vitality squares yourself, and you find how to discharge them yourself, there is no compelling reason to contract a Reiki Master to recuperate you. Since you can do it without anyone else's help. The best job a Reiki Master can take is spurring you to change. Since without change, there is no genuine advancement. The vitality of Reiki itself will help change to happen naturally. Anyway, by learning Reiki, you enable that change to turn out to be a lot further and unquestionably increasingly significant.

Chapter 4: Getting Started: Your Self-Healing Process

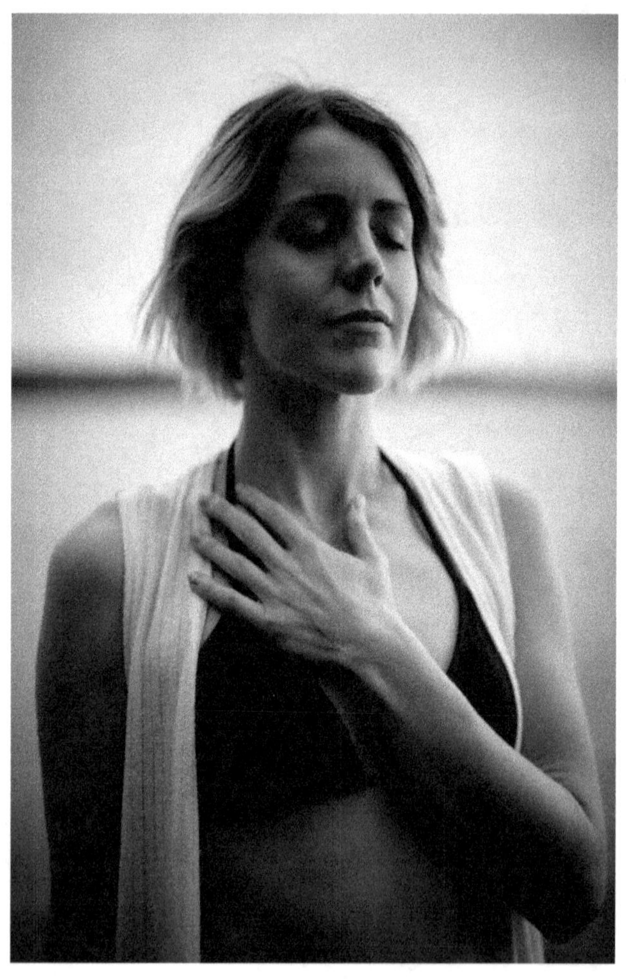

A Brief Introduction to Self-Healing

Every one of us comes into this presentation with an exceptional arrangement of individual characteristics that incorporate aptitudes that can form into abilities and capacities. Likewise, there are regularly testing circumstances that influence us. Like the rudder on a pontoon, our decisions figure out what course we take throughout everyday life and what conceivable outcomes we investigate and create. When we are gone up against troubles, just as circumstances, it is the way we manage them that decides how they influence us. So, it is significant that we utilize our capacity to pick astutely. An actual existence all around lived is an existence of development or an existence of recuperating and improvement.

As we think back on our lives, it is anything but difficult to see defining moments where we settled on a decision that powerfully affected where our life went and who we moved toward becoming. By pondering our past decisions and where they have taken us, it is conceivable to gain from our encounters and improve our capacity to pick. Life is loaded up with numerous conceivable outcomes, and it is imperative to understand that occasionally it is the more troublesome choice that presents to us the best advantage.

In the event that you are sick in any capacity or in the event that you are encountering any piece of your life that is not as much as what you might want, realize that it is conceivable to change, to recuperate, and to make the sort of life you need. In the event that you need something you don't have, at that point the most significant thing you have to do is to pick this for yourself. At that point make a move.

The universe is consistently in a condition of parity. An issue, trouble or testing circumstance can't exist except if its answer exists simultaneously. In the event that you need to take care of an issue, the main thing you should do is to conclude that you are going to discover the arrangement.

Here is a law of the psyche, a law of life that is critical to get it. Definiteness of direction continued after some time consistently creates results. Consider this: it generally creates results. This is the most significant idea you can concentrate on as far or as close to home in terms of recuperating and achievement. In the event that you need to recuperate, you have to shape this into a clear reason and seek after it with energy and remain with it until you are mended.

The brain resembles a magnet. It pulls in its opinion of most, the more grounded the considerations the more grounded the fascination. On the off chance that you need to mend yourself, or build up any positive quality, it is significant for you to make an obvious choice this is the thing that you will do. As you hold this idea in your brain with the positive conviction, and knowingness that you will accomplish your outcome, you will draw into yourself every one of the assets and individuals you have to make the outcomes you need.

We each have extraordinary gifts, characteristics and diamonds of significant worth that we may not be completely communicating or maybe not communicating by any means. We were conceived on this planet to satisfy a reason and that object is to find our reality, what our identity is, the thing that makes us interesting, claim this valuable piece of ourselves and express it to the world.

Self-Healing Program

In building up your own Reiki self-recuperating program it is imperative to require some investment to attempt various strategies. As you do as such, know about the outcomes and if the system is by all accounts pushing you toward your objective. In the event that it is, proceed with it. On the off chance that it isn't, have a go at something different. Along these lines, you will build up an individual arrangement of mending that is actually directly for you. This will significantly improve your outcomes. There are numerous approaches to utilize Reiki and I might want to display a couple of thoughts and strategies that are amazing and powerful.

Self-Treatments

Utilization of self-medicines is a significant piece of any Reiki mending/personal development program. Put aside 15 to 30 minutes every day to give yourself a Reiki treatment. This can be a finished treatment utilizing all the hand positions or you could utilize Boysen checking and treat just those territories you are guided to. While giving yourself Reiki, your vibration will go up and as this happens, I propose you enable yourself to examine the different exercises occurring in your life. As you do this, all things considered, you will discover sound new frames of mind creating about issues throughout your life, just as get inventive thoughts on the most proficient method to manage them. So as to monitor this, I propose you get a scratchpad to compose these thoughts in and afterward use them in your activity plans.

Individual Healing Alliance

Getting medications from others is additionally significant and truth be told, this is likely the most significant thing you can do to keep your Reiki vitality solid. We propose you go above and beyond and build up an individual recuperating partnership. To do this, discover somebody you can believe who additionally has a wellbeing or life issue they need to mend. Meet at any rate once per week to trade Reiki sessions and offer what has occurred since your last gathering. Structure an understanding between you and how you will bolster each other totally in discovering answers for your issues and ending up totally recuperated. Be eager to share everything and keep what you share in your gatherings carefully private. Utilize all the imagination and motivation that surfaces to understand your issues or accomplish your objectives. During the week put aside time to send far off Reiki to one another. You can likewise call each other on the telephone if something comes up. These gatherings must be paid attention to and it is imperative to concentrate on the means recorded above and not enable them to slip into only a get-together. This is an exceptionally incredible procedure and will bring profound and extremely important degrees of recuperating.

Reiki Affirmations and Prayers

Reiki can be utilized in an amazing manner to upgrade insistences and supplications. Spot your recuperating objective or wanted achievement on a 3x5 card. Utilizing vitality, draw Reiki images over the card. We suggest utilizing each of the three Reiki II images and any others you may have. At that point hold the card between your hands and give the card Reiki. As you do as such, rehash your insistence as well as state a supplication offering gratitude that your objective has been accomplished or that your mending has occurred. State your attestation as well as supplication again and again. Do this with conviction in any event once per day. You can likewise convey the card with you and rehash this procedure at whatever point you have an extra minute during the day.

Going Against the Issue

A procedure that will quicken recuperating is to conflict with the issue and use Reiki to mend the sentiments and energies that surface. On the off chance that you have a dread of accomplishing something, feel free to do it in any case - conflict with the dread. This procedure stimulates torpid mental emotions making them rise to the top where you can all the more effectively utilize your Reiki to mend or discharge them. It takes fortitude, yet it is ground-breaking. Have a Reiki companion work with you to help if conceivable. For instance, on the off chance that you have a dread of open talking, feel free to organize to give a discourse. Before the discourse give yourself Reiki, and spotlight on any sentiments that are coming up. After and notwithstanding during the discourse, give yourself Reiki concentrating on the sentiments. Or then again, on the off chance that you have a dread of gathering individuals, choose to go to a gathering and intentionally acquaint yourself with individuals at the gathering. Give yourself Reiki previously, after and during the gathering if conceivable. In the event that it is excessively startling to physically do it, at that point simply envision doing it in your psyche and direct Reiki to the out of this world and up. In the wake of treating the issue along these lines, sooner or later you will have the option to do it seriously. When utilizing this procedure, it is critical to utilize good judgment and not take part in any exercises that could be perilous.

Raising Your Vibration

Anything that will raise your vibration will enable you to mend all the more rapidly. Doing things; for example, improving your nourishment, building up an activity program, reflection, getting sufficient rest and rest, knead, yoga activities or extending, Tai Chi, social exercises and different types of excitement will act to raise your vibration. As your vibration goes up, it will be simpler for you to pick up understanding into your circumstance and make progressively viable arrangements. It will likewise make every single other type of recuperating work better.

Utilization of Other Modalities

Keep in mind that Reiki works in a positive manner with every other type of recuperating. In this way, with your unmistakable expectation, and the utilization of Reiki vitality you might be guided to other mending assets. Be watchful for these extra recuperating techniques. Strategies; for example, different systems, changes in eating routine, the utilization of herbs, and homeopathic cures, and so forth. These could incredibly improve your recuperating procedure.

Therapeutic and Psychological Care

There are numerous superb medicinal specialists and analysts who are available to elective mending. In the event that you have a restorative or mental condition, it is significant that you get their recommendation and tail it on the off chance that you feel guided to do as such. On the off chance that you have a genuine condition and medical procedure, or medications are suggested, it is essential to get a subsequent supposition before choosing what to do. Keep in mind, Reiki works in concordance with drug and brain research and there might be some significant and even vital treatments they can offer. It is imperative to think about them when building up your recuperating program.

These are a couple of approaches to utilize Reiki to make your own recuperating program. Your inward direction and your reasonable goal will make you find others not referenced here. Being completely occupied with this procedure is important in the event that you are to determine the best advantage. To cite Helen Keller, "Life is an exciting adventure or nothing at all." You are the person who chooses what direction it will be for you. The difficulties we face in life contain the exercises we are here to learn. Try not to pull back from them, nor endeavor to settle them indifferently, however rather, completely grasp them. Achievement of a commendable close to home objective carries with it something beyond the outcomes you were searching for. It additionally brings the specific learning that we can change and make the sort of life we need. At last, when we inspect our lives, it isn't so much what we know in our minds that is significant, nor even what we do but what we become.

Practice Meditation

Simply put, meditation is the supercharging of our spiritual battery, just as sleep charges our physical battery, except that eight hours for meditation are not required. Meditation removes barriers that our imagination creates. It is the place to go for answers to the most intimate problems. It is non-judgmental and is free of charge. Pressure from everyday living can make us want to throw our hands up, give up and not try, or give up and quit trying, saying " I can' t do this on my own. I need help."

Meditation practice is many thousands of years old, handed down from numerous Eastern cultures such as Hindu, Chinese, Korean, Indonesian, and Japanese. Meditation is the art of becoming still and quietening the mind, silence the monkey-mind bandit, and commune with spirit to unleash infinite cosmic resources and capabilities, so that we may reach our best and better- yet experience.

In his Book of Essays by Ralph Waldo Emerson, the author and philosopher adroitly expresses the importance of meditation in the chapter The Over-Soul:

" There is a difference between one and another hour of life in their authority and subsequent effect···Man is a stream whose source is hidden. Always our being is descending into us from we know not whence···As with events, so it is with thoughts. When I watch the flowing river, which out of regions I see not, pours for a season its streams into me – I see that I am a pensioner – not a cause but a surprised spectator of this ethereal water; that I desire and look up and put myself in the attitude of reception..."

Translated, in one hour a person can morph in his or her stream of thought from despair to soaring with eagles; one can evolve from enslavement to ideas of lack, glass ceilings, bad luck, clinging to possessions or people, and re-living victim situations, to relax into the rhythm of flowing nature where all is well and in perfect order. Water is the carrier of life without which life cannot thrive. World famous Astrophysicist, Dr. Neil deGrasse Tyson tells us that we are all made of star stuff. Everything in existence is all made from the same basic elements. What a unifying thought, that we are all one with each other – sisters and brothers with everything and everyone that exists – the stars and planets, the Moon, the Sun, volcanoes and glaciers and icebergs; predator beasts on land and the fish in the sea, the birds in the air, the flowing river – our neighbors up and down the street – and distant nations around the globe! Metaphysically water represents consciousness, that fertile place in the Mind which nurtures whatever seeds of thought are planted there and will grow into life experience. This cosmic river' s source is unknown yet ever flowing, and so is ours. As it relates to chakra meditation, C.W. Leadbeater notes:

" In body meditation the region of water is declared to extend from the knees to the anus. The water is semi-lunar in shape and white in color"

Contemplating the river's surface, dazzled by its shimmering beauty, breathing in fully, I gently guide my breath to the root chakra and blend with the river's flow, and I am transported in thought, delving far beneath the surface to explore my subconscious mind where immense possibilities await my discovery! Trust and surrender equals peace.

Monkey-mind is the chatter we engage ourselves in when we're at a neutral, non-working unoccupied with chores place in our mental and physical processes; commuting, showering, preparing meals, catching up on the latest news or family gossip. It's that fertile space in our mind which takes up problems, worries, doubts, insecurities, jealousies, and remembers something somebody said to tick you off. And once the monkey-mind door is open the negativity floods right in like a deluge. It will stay there if you don't arrest it and put it where it belongs – OUT! Consistent, daily meditation strengthens spiritual awareness and helps keep monkey chatter at bay, guides the subconscious mind to absorb and assimilate the Mind of Infinity, Divine Mind.

Charles Fillmore, author, minister and co-founder of Unity Ministries wrote in his book entitled Prosperity:

" Divine Mind is the one and only reality. When we

incorporate the ideas that form this Mind into our mind and persevere in those ideas, a mighty strength wells up within us…When the spiritual body is established in consciousness, its strength and power is transmitted to the visible body and to all the things that we touch in the world around us."
Prosperity is thriving. It is success demonstrated as good health, mutually respectful relationships at home, at work doing work we love, and at play. It is rich self-esteem that is not boastful or haughty. And it is financial well-being. Prosperity is promised in the hand of anyone holding an American dollar bill. In fact, " E pluribus Unum," the Latin phrase on American currency means " One in many."
" Mind substance enters into every little detail of your daily life whether you realize the Truth or not."
The beginning of meditation is around 15,000 years ago with Shiva. It is written that Shiva (Adiyogi) the Lord of Meditation was the first guru of yoga extoling meditation in universal consciousness. He was a cosmic dancer who danced ecstatically on the Himalayas. Enlightened, he possessed an active third eye which enables intuition and spiritual mastery. The Hindu practice of Jhana has been known as " the training of the mind" since 1500 BC. And in China, from 600 to 300 BC the Daoist Laozi described such meditation practices as:

Shou Zhong – "guarding the middle",

Bao Yi – "embracing the one",

Shou Jing – "guarding tranquility", and

Bao Pu "embracing simplicity",

Zen – "dhyana" Meditation Japanese Sanskrit 12th century.

There are many meditation disciplines and techniques, among them are:

Buddhist Meditation: based on the principles of Buddhism to develop concentration, clarity, and calmness; focuses on the breath

Chakra Meditation: first century Tantric tradition guiding and training the breath, and light visualization within each chakra. Training the breath to circulate and invigorate the vital energy at specific chakra areas for healing or for energy balance

Loving-Kindness Meditation: also called Metta meditation; to foster an attitude of love and compassion toward everything including adversaries and causes of tension; self-guided active image meditation

Mindfulness Meditation: created by Dr. Jon Kabat-Zin, professor of medicine, during the 1970s; focusing on thoughts, emotions and sensations in the present moment

Mahamudra Meditation: rooted in India, it has been

practiced in order to capture the transparency and essential accuracy of the mind

Raja Yoga Meditation: first mentioned in the Bhagavad Gita, with eyes open focus on an object; benefits are understanding the importance of silence and introspection, improves clarity and concentration

Shiva Meditation: Practice opens the third eye, enables your mind to function in the highest possible manner in perception and understanding

Transcendental Meditation: also known as TM was introduced by Maharishi Mahesh Yogi in the mid-1950s; technique is to silently repeat a mantra, which is given the participant according to age and gender, is practiced to still the mind

Vipassana Meditation: an ancient Buddhist discipline of continued attention to sensation to gain mindfulness and insight.

Zen Meditation: from Chinese Buddhism brought to Japan by a South Indian king, based in spirituality, relieves stress and relaxes, aids in solving core problems and making wiser decisions.

The list is not complete. There are several other meditation practices from which to choose. Why choose Chakra meditation?

In Chakra meditation each one of the seven chakras brings its own qualities and characteristics. To breathe, prana, into a particular chakra carries life sustaining oxygen, air and water specifically to that area to vivify all five aspects of the person (astral, spiritual, mental, psychological, and physical) and to stimulate whole-self healing in the entire person. Breathing into the heart chakra for example, will increase its undulating activity to brighten the energy charge and exude more strength in awakening according to the law of attraction; to love, to grow and to prosper.

The key is concentrating on the breath. Breathing into the solar plexus for example, the Navel chakra will stimulate the law of attraction and stimulate enthusiasm, success, clarity, and aid to balance the will power in the individual.

There are various other meditation techniques that focus on the breath, and several require concentration on something, either visually with eyes open, or with the imagination. Some are audibly guided by a group leader; others are self-guided. Chakra meditation can be done alone or with a guide.

The results of meditation are subtle and if you are not looking closely, you can miss out on small transitions as they are happening. Let' s say for example, you' ve been in the habit of biting your nails all your life. You make a lifestyle change and start meditating consistently on a daily basis.

One day you notice that you need a manicure because your nails are so long you can' t type comfortably on your keyboard anymore. Congratulations!

How to Get Started

To start any Reiki practice, you should enact the vitality inside yourself. Close your eyes and take a couple of rounds of full breaths. Envision the crown of your head opening and a flood of mending white light spilling out of the highest point of your head, into your heart, and out through your arms and hands. Request to be topped off where you need recuperating most. Along these lines, in case you're going to offer Reiki to a friend or family member, you won't give them from an unfilled cup.

As you feel the progression of vitality, proceed to inhale, and on the off chance that you discover your brain gets occupied or begins to address whether this is working, returned to your breath. Imagine yourself as a vessel for mending. At that point set an expectation or petition to get recuperating of the most noteworthy great.

To give a rest centered Reiki session to a companion or relative, request that the beneficiary rests while you position yourself close to their head.
Envision a constant flow of mending light going from your

hands into the back of their head and clearing the brain of any agony or uneasiness encountered that day.

Request that your cherished one take a few rounds of full breaths and gradually tally a breath in of three seconds and breathe out of three to five seconds.

Ask them to gradually observe the entirety of their very first-moment memory at once and to thank every memory before releasing it with their breath.

Enable them to float off as you keep on directing the vitality through your palms and send the recuperating light into their whole body. Envision the body getting to be mended, loose, and overwhelming for a serene night's rest. You can offer this Reiki for whatever length of time that you need, however somewhere in the range of fifteen and thirty minutes is generally enough for them to feel loose and tranquil.

Regularly when individuals have tension and stress, they are not breathing appropriately, and the brevity of breath can cause more pressure. In this Reiki session, you need to channel vitality down the beneficiary's shoulders and into their body. Spot your hands on their shoulders for ten to fifteen minutes. Concentrate on sending vitality into their entire body and breathing profoundly with them. This can normally bring a portion of the extraordinary mental vitality down and get them again into their body. In the event that your individual is resting, you can put your hands behind their head, as well, to enable them to quiet down.

It's imperative to offer appreciation, purge yourself, and close the vitality once you've finished a recuperating session. It very well may be as straightforward as venturing back, cleaning your hands of any abundance vitality, and putting them in supplication to express gratitude toward yourself, the vitality, and the beneficiary for the trade. You can likewise draw an enormous circle, crossing the arms before the body to mean the end of your two energies and closure with hands in the petition.

In case you're offering Reiki to your accomplice or different grown-ups, recollect that a few grown-ups, after some time, have overlooked how to feel (or have turned out to be less mindful of) their fiery and physical body. That is alright. Simply realize that they may state that they can't feel the vitality moving. It may be unobtrusive, yet it doesn't imply that your vitality didn't influence them.

When working with children, contingent upon their age, it can likewise impart to them what you are doing and why. Children are keen and will, in general, be unimaginably open to elective practices. A few guardians will likewise tell kids the best way to get vitality and do Reiki themselves, so they start to get to their entry to mending at an early age.

Practicing Reiki on Yourself: Finding Happiness from Within

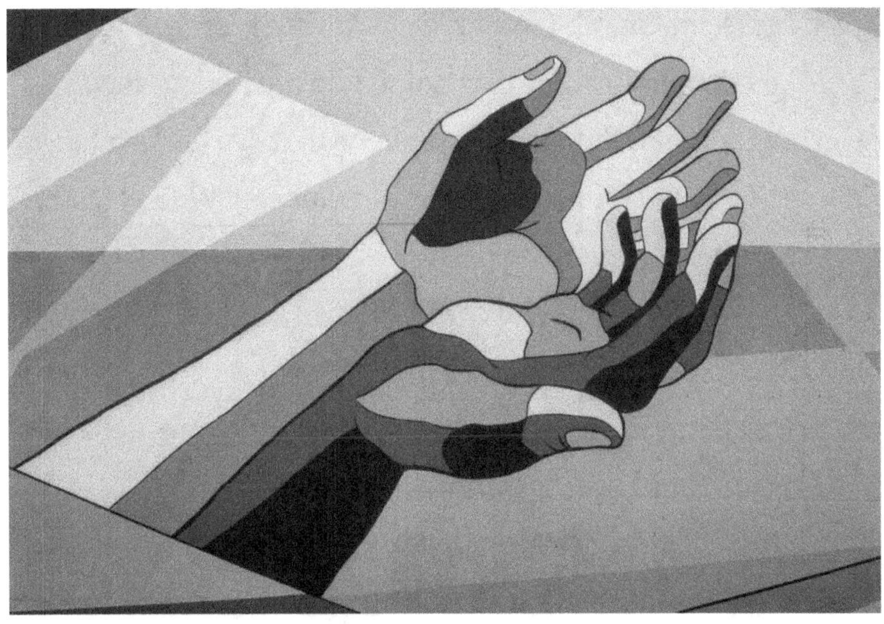

Reiki works best in the event that you maintain things simple and straightforward.

The longest rehearsing Master of Reiki in the Western world, John Harvey Gray, and who carried on with a solid and dynamic life into his nineties practiced Reiki by teaming it up with self-recuperating process for an extended period of time.

"During the evening I do my head and my neck, my eyes, the side of my head that has to do with hearing and my throat. On the off chance that I have had an especially enthusiastic day or on the off chance that I wake up and can't return to rest, I place my hands behind my head. We typically do that around evening time. At that point, I do my middle toward the beginning of the day. In the event that I've had a major dinner, I do my stomach area to help digest it. When I get an irritated throat, which happens rarely, I'll do five or six hours on my sinuses, throat, and chest. Once in a while, I treat my liver. We treat any situation as meager or as much as I need to since I know where my wellbeing difficulties are. Reiki for self-recuperating is a powerful pressure. We are a substantially more serene individual now than when I was in the business world. We are a lot more beneficial than I would have been in the event that I had not learned and drilled Reiki. I've outlasted the normal age for men in my family and hope to keep living longer and healthy."

Regularly, individuals become profoundly loose when performing Reiki for their own healing and subsequently doze off. It should be noted that there is nothing wrong with that. Appreciate resting after having attained a deep state of relaxation. Reiki can be done at any time such as when you are in a deep sleep, while watching television, at the moment you are sitting down in a chair or in a meeting room, while driving down the road, or while hanging tight for the dental specialist or a business arrangement to begin. Simply rest your hands any place you need the recuperating vitality and it will stream, discreetly and subtly, even while you are snoozing.

Start your more joyful, more advantageous life by fusing these Reiki-based systems:

Set a caution on your watch or telephone each hour for eight hours. Respite for three minutes and notice things around you. Notice hues, temperature, individuals and quietness. Focus on anything in your condition. On the off chance that you think that it's difficult to know about the things around, you start straightforward. Wash your dishes as opposed to thudding them in the dishwasher.
Notice the water temperature, the air pockets and the fragrance of the cleanser. This activity causes you to know about your environment and eventually you become mindful of yourself in your environment.

You don't need to wear a robe, go to a mountain or sit in a

pretzel position to think. Reflection intends to focus your full focus on a solitary thing. The purpose of contemplation is to calm your psyche. Logical research demonstrates that reflection diminishes the battle/flight reaction causing an abatement in pulse and circulatory strain, which is heart solid! To rehearse reflection, locate a tranquil spot where you won't be aggravated —even a restroom slow down can work and take a couple of minutes to take eight full breaths and spotlight on something you can consider such to be a door handle or tree.

Penelope Quest says, "Your feelings can manage you, yet you don't need to give them a chance to control you." If you get yourself fast to outrage or are commonly irate, you have shaped a propensity to respond to circumstances with annoyance.

Nonetheless, you can change your responses. You can utilize running, strolling and breathing as prompt approaches to diminish your annoyance and help change the manner in which you respond.A long-haul strategy is to reconstruct your responses; for example, perceptual positions. Notice "oneself" first. Notice what you hear, feel and see. At that point attempt to be the other individual in the circumstance. Notice what they see, hear and feel. Presently, be an onlooker and notice what you would see, hear and feel as somebody standing close by.

You've heard, "For getting healthy, the kind of food you eat is everything" and the equivalent is valid for "you are what you think." Try this: Stand in the mirror and rehash the words "I am tragic" multiple times. Notice what befalls your stance —drooping shoulders, head drops, breathing changes. Presently rehash "I am upbeat" multiple times. See what befalls your non-verbal communication and relaxing. Discover a word each week to rehash to yourself in the mirror. Make a rundown of your characteristics: great cook, great mother, keen companion, great competitor, etc.

Start your day offering gratitude for five things throughout your life. In case you're having an unpleasant time seeing something as appreciative for, start with the climate. Express appreciation for downpour or daylight. Do this consistently and soon it will be a programmed procedure.

Additionally, practice otherworldly wellness to be more grounded, clear and merciful. In an ordinary circumstance; for example, meeting a companion for lunch, question the motivation behind why you've been allowed the chance to share time together. Locate the higher motivation behind the circumstances and openings you are given. Another approach to practice otherworldly wellness is to make a rundown of 10 things that fulfill you. Do something consistently.

Guided Reiki Self-Session

In spite of the fact that it is a superb encounter to get Reiki from another person, a companion or an expert, there are numerous motivations to consider figuring out how to rehearse Reiki on yourself.
The accommodation of self-care is esteemed by individuals with wellbeing challenges, yet additionally by others with occupied calendars who are looking for more parity in their lives.

Everyday Reiki self-care gives a chance to reestablish harmony, lessen pressure, and reconnect with an encounter of health.

Furthermore, snapshots of Reiki practice for the duration of the day can bring focusing and alleviation from agony, tension, and worry as regularly as required. Individuals experiencing uneasiness or agony who learn Reiki self-care have the extra strengthening of realizing they are never again alone and vulnerable with their torment.

Learning Reiki self-care can profit individuals who are solid and those with incessant wellbeing conditions, regardless of whether it's diabetes, asthma, malignancy, epilepsy, weakness disorders, wretchedness, or coronary illness, to give some examples. They can rehearse Reiki on themselves consistently to decrease pressure and fortify prosperity and rehash the Reiki practice as regularly as they feel the need.

There is additionally some narrative proof that Reiki has the potential for profiting creatures in a significant number of similar ways experienced by people. Those offering Reiki to their pets are regularly wonderfully shocked at their pet's advantage and collaboration!

At the point when there are budgetary confinements, the benefits of a one-time interest in figuring out how to rehearse Reiki self-care overpaying for rehashed sessions are self-evident. At the point when there is a disease in a family and it is never again practical for the patient to self-treat, at least one relative can adapt First degree (hands-on) Reiki and treat the patient and other relatives just as themselves.

You can just take in Reiki from a certified Reiki ace. One approach to discover a Reiki ace is to ask companions that training Reiki with whom they contemplated. You can likewise solicit neighborhood experts from other correlative treatments; for example, a back rub or shiatsu, in light of the fact that these specialists frequently know other reciprocal treatment suppliers.

On the other hand, you can check notice sheets in yoga studios and wellbeing nourishment stores or ask if your nearby clinic has a corresponding or integrative prescription administration. Since numerous individuals to adapt to incessant ailment utilize Reiki, any nearby association that offers administrations to individuals with diseases; for example, malignancy, HIV, fibromyalgia, or diabetes may have a rundown of network assets.

It is critical to take note of that Reiki is certainly not an institutionalized practice thus there is no assurance that anybody utilizing the title "Reiki ace" has the preparation and experience you look for in an instructor/guide. Thus, it's critical to ask into any Reiki ace's experience, and a trustworthy Reiki ace will respect this request.

Furthermore, make certain to get some information about the Reiki ace's showing knowledge and classes (planning, expense, and so on). Lastly, ask what openings the Reiki ace ideas for kept coaching and gathering practice. Pick your Reiki ace cautiously, looking not just for an instructor who has the capabilities you need; yet, in addition for one with whom you feel compatibility.

Hand Positioning in Self-Treatment

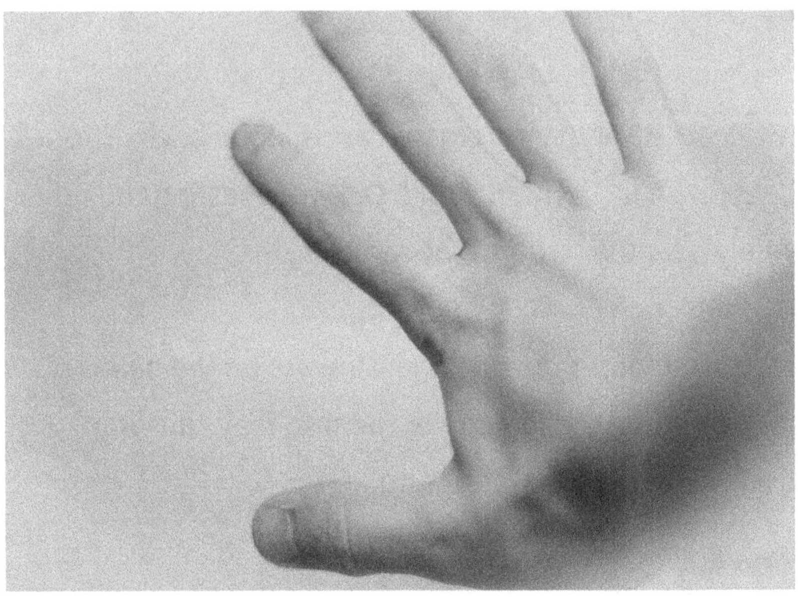

There are twelve fundamental hand arrangements for the most part utilized when giving yourself a Reiki treatment. These hand positions are not unchangeable; yet, rather, fill in as a rule for new understudies behaving medications. They are likewise useful in utilizing to lead a one-hour recuperating session. Apply five minutes for every position.

Face: Place your palms upon your face, setting them gently upon your eyes and fingers thus transforming them into a sanctuary. No weight required - contact delicately!

Top of Head and Crown: Locate hands to the opposite positions of the head, the set down hand gently close to the ears. Then, with your fingertips, reach out for the top of your head.

Back of Head: After having crossed arms at the back of your head, set one hand behind your head while resting the other peacefully over the scruff of the neck.

Jawline and chin: Set down the jaw inward on the palms of your deliberate hands, empower them so they can wrap alongside all of the facial structure.

Heart and collarbone: The neck should be serenely grabbed from the inside of your thumb and fingers which ought to be forming a " V" shape. Your hand should be lowered down and it should rest in between your heart center and the collarbone.

Midsection and Rib Cage: Set hands on your ribs, on the upper section, keep clearly underneath your chest. Extricate up elbows in a flexed position.

Waist: Upon your stomach, set hands (the section known as " solar plexus") over the belly button, empowering the tips of your fingers to contact.

Pelvis: Set a hand on opposite sides of the pelvic bones, empowering the tips of your fingers for touch.

Shoulder blades: Place arms on top of your head, elbows bowed, and hands placed over your shoulder blades. Then again, set hands over your shoulder bones if you can't land at your shoulder bones effectively.

Midback: For the midback position, reach regardless of your great confidence with bowed elbows and set hands on the convergence point of the back.

Lower Back: Next hands circumstances are on the lower back. Reach in spite of your great confidence, elbows bowed and with your hands placed on the lower region of the back.

Sacrum: The last hand position is the sacrum. Place your hands further down in order to recognize the sacral section with the hands.

Western Style Self-Treatment

More data has become exposed in the course of the most recent couple of years that give a decent comprehension of the History of Reiki. The Reiki we know as Shin-Shin Kaizen Usui Reiki Ryoho might have been 'found' by Mikao Usui subsequent to achieving illumination after a mountain retreat on Mount Kurama in March 1922. He began this fasting as planning for death. He did this for 20 or more days and felt an amazing vitality stun on his temple and wound up oblivious. He was in this state for a couple of hours anyway when he returned to cognizance, he felt shockingly new and empowered more than he had previously. Reiki vitality had entered his body and soul and had the acknowledgment that 'The Universe is me-I am the Universe.'

Usui sensei was conceived on fifteenth August 1865 in Taniamura, Yamagata-firearm, Gifu. He had different professions including a secretary to a statesman that gave him numerous encounters and a point of view of the world from numerous edges. He delighted in movement in his childhood and this drove him to think about the inquiry 'What is the motivation behind life'. He contemplated a wide range of subjects including Buddhism, Psychology, and Christianity to give some examples. After much investigation, he reached the resolution that 'a definitive reason forever is to achieve A Jin-Ryu-Mei – the condition of complete genuine feelings of serenity.

This drove him to think about Zen Buddhism and in the long run to his excursion to Mount Kurama.

After his illumination, he kept running down the mountain and stubbed his toe, subsequent to lying on his hands he found the torment vanished and his toe mended. From this, he began to lay hands on others and discovered this began to mend loved ones. This drove him to systemize this as the Reiki we know today.

He set up his very own establishment 'Usui Reiki Ryoho Gakkai' when he moved to Aoyama-Harajuku in Tokyo. From that point, he began leading workshops and educating individuals.

Reiki spread broadly and when Japan was hit with the Earthquake in 1923 the requirement for Reiki as of now was clear with a huge number harmed, so Reiki turned out to be amazingly famous. Usui sensei kicked the bucket in 1926 after three strokes, it is accounted for that he was giving Reiju at the time. It is thought he realized he was going to bite the dust so started 20 Dai Shihans to guarantee Reiki proceeded after his demise.

One of his most noticeable understudies was Chujiro Hayashi sensei and when he was 47 in finished all degrees of Reiki (Shoden, Okuden, and Shinpiden) – this was only preceding Usui Sensei biting the dust. He was a maritime official and a medicinal specialist and rehearsed Reiki in Shinano-machi Tokyo. He educated Reiki in Osaka just as Tokyo and included Hawayo Takata who was a Japanese American conceived in Hawaii who truly began the spread of Reiki toward the West and the remainder of the World.

Hayashi sensei gave Reiki classes in Hawaii to 5 months between October 1937 and February 1938.

Hawayo Takata ended up intrigued and began to learn through a correspondence course with Hayashi Sensei in Tokyo. This is believed to be a trade of letters and through her eagerness she got an endorsement to head out to Tokyo around December 1935 to learn. She prepared for a half year and it is thought she was endorsed as a Shihankaku when she left Japan. She showed 50 individuals Shoden while as yet relating with Hayashi Sensei.

In July 1937 she returned to Japan and finished her preparation and was offered an endorsement to be a Shihan. Hayashi Sensei then touched base in Hawaii where in 5 months he showed a sum of 350 understudies. Hawayo Takata facilitated his visit and proceeded with the workshops after he left.

The subsequent World War cast a shadow over Reiki, and it took Hawayo Takata 40 years to continue the exercises to advance Reiki in Hawaii. She started preparing instructors around 1978 and by 1980 when she kicked the bucket had shown 22 of them.

Reiki spread immediately when it went to terrain America and from that point to the entire world.

In the mid-1990's Reiki was 'reintroduced' to Japan; yet, educated by Western instructors. So, in influence from the Hawayo Takata heredity and not immediate from Chujiro Hayashi sensei. Jikiden Reiki started its voyage after Chiyoko Yamaguchi's Uncle Wasaburo Sugano who got Reiju from Hayashi Sensei and turning into a Reiki expert treating family, companions, and associates. Chiyoko lived with the family and was dealt with like his little girl. Sugano was a noteworthy supporter of making Reiki prominent and he asked Hayashi Sensei to hold a workshop in Ishikawa, on the stipulation that there would be in excess of 10 participants.

In the family, Reiki was drilled day by day and Chiyoko was constantly dazzled and felt better after been dealt with. She once in a while expected to see a specialist so was constantly quick to learn herself, her Uncle bolstered this however simply after she moved on from school. She was just 17 when she went to the workshop of Shoden and Okuden on thirteenth March 1938. She was anxious and energized and was one of the more youthful participants close by more established men in formal clothing. She noticed the 3 columns of 6 Zabuton (Japanese style pads) on the floor and was approached to sit on them.

The facilitator running the occasion at that point clarified the Reiju and how it was finished. Taking note of that the room would be obscured and understudies ought to sit in Seiza pose with eyes shut setting hands in Gassho. There was to be no talking or leaving the seat until after Reiju.

Hayashi sensei then went into the room and the room was dull. He began by discussing the Gokai and the understudies rehashed line by line multiple times. They were then given Reiju first by Hayashi Sensei and afterward the others. Chiyoko assessed there were 3 Shihans yet wasn't certain as it was dull and each Reiju took around 5 minutes. There pursued the Reiki Mawashi. Hayashi Sensei then proceeded to clarify the hypothesis of Reiki before training on others and sentiment of vitality. So, this was Chiyoko's first understanding of Reiju and Jikiden Reiki pursues that equivalent configuration today.

With the reintroduction of Reiki to Japan, it was the

Westernized Lineage Reiki been instructed. Anyway, a couple of individuals attempted to follow the roots of Reiki in Japan; however, the Usui Reiki Ryoho Gakkai is shut to the overall population and the first lessons do not happen. So, it was hard to perceive how the first type of Reiki educated be Usui sensei and Hayashi Sensei could be scholarly.

Tadao and Chiyoko were utilizing Reiki consistently unconscious of the prominence of Reiki and that individuals were looking for data. In 1999 Chiyoko was referenced in a book composed by a well-known educator in Japan and massively affected the Reiki people group. There was an interest that they had found somebody instructed straightforwardly from Hayashi sensei and as yet rehearsing every day following 65 years.

After the production of the book, Chiyoko was visited by noticeable Reiki instructors who suggested running workshops that recreated those held by Hayashi sensei. In the wake of catching a discussion that Reiki was no major ordeal, Tadao was told the substance of the workshop. They had gone though he was flabbergasted at how far expelled it was from the Reiki soul he held. It caused him to acknowledge that it was so essential to pass on the first

Hayashi sensei lessons. It was then chosen to begin the Jikiden Reiki Kenkyukai and workshops.

Self-Treatment for Areas Difficult to Reach

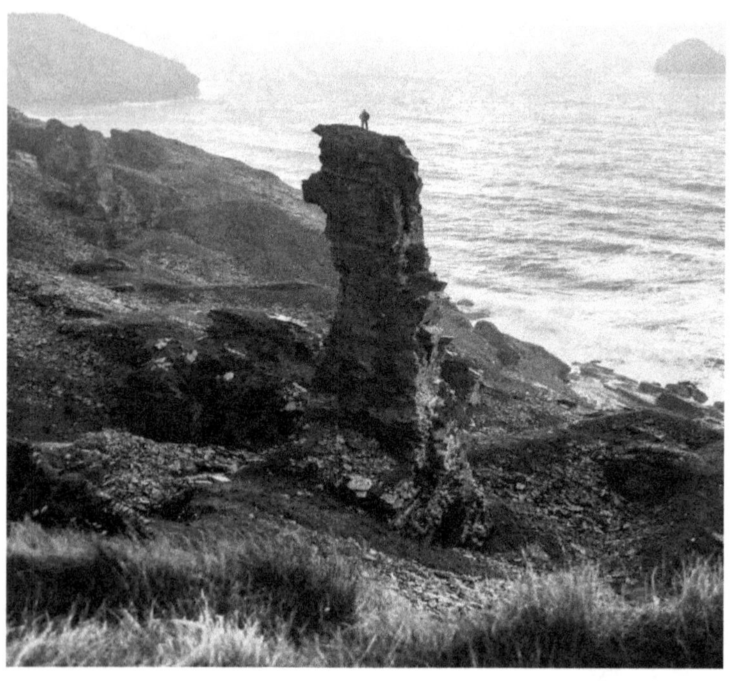

Reiki resembles a muscle. The more you use it, the more grounded it might turn into. Also, utilizing Reiki on yourself day by day is only one approach to improve your inward Reiki practice. Here come seven additional procedures that can enable you to improve your training and beat difficulties.

In uncommon situations when experts may feel like their Reiki vitality isn't as energetic not surprisingly, they could be encountering a vitality stagnation or square in their frameworks for some explanation, as life happens to everybody. While self-Reiki is an amazingly valuable device for keeping the vitality solid, getting hands-on Reiki from others additionally can be an incredible answer for assistance unblock and renew dormant vitality.

Reiki urges one's own mending to occur, with specialists only filling in as vessels through which the vitality streams. At the point when experts become excessively vested in the result of treating an especially dear companion or relative, they may overlook that Reiki and that individual's higher self is in control. This can leave the expert with weakness. Relinquish the result and let Reiki do its work. As a wise recuperating vitality, it knows precisely where to go, what to do and how to do it.

Reiki is certainly not a vicious field loaded with enough challenge. In the event that your passion rises when more Reiki experts or administrations touch base in your general vicinity, take a full breath and be appreciative.

Be appreciative an ever-increasing number of individuals are getting to be intrigued and associated with Reiki.

Remember there is a lot more prominent requirement for mending than there are Reiki experts who can offer it. Your very own training is progressively able to stay steady and solid in the event that you invite other Reiki specialists with an open heart.

In the event that you accept your Reiki business will come up short, there's a decent shot it will. Really and unequivocally trust it will flourish, and there's a decent possibility it will. The brain resembles a goliath magnet that draws as a general rule that matches your contemplations. Choose you will make an effective Reiki practice that you are deserving of doing as such and the numerous individuals you advantage will effortlessly exceed any difficulties you experience making it.

In case you're rehearsing Reiki in a narrow-minded manner, with your solitary objective as profiting or picking up control or eminence, at that point you're probably going to have an extreme time building up a flourishing practice. You may have a much harder time getting help from your soul aides, holy messengers and your own higher self that could some way or another help with customers and your general practice. Return to your goal, guaranteeing it has a solid profound premise, and these higher wellsprings of assistance might be promptly accessible to aid any way they can.

Keeping your Reiki vitality solid, your goal profound and benevolence in your heart goes far toward improving any Reiki practice. For whatever length of time that you likewise make sure to deal with different parts of your being. This should be possible with sufficient rest, a sound eating routine, adjusted remaining burden and setting aside an effort to take part in different exercises that you appreciate; for example, contemplation, yoga, practice and, above all, an everyday portion of appreciation.

The possibility that spirits can be the reason for sick wellbeing and different issues has been a typical conviction among healers since antiquated occasions. Jesus was said to recuperate by throwing out spirits, also, present-day healers keep on working with that misinformed spirits could cause issues. Plenty of procedures exist to discharge spirits, which differ in its level of adequacy. We might want to depict a strategy utilizing Reiki that is both safe and exceptionally compelling. This system can be utilized to discharge a soul from an individual or from an area; for example, a home. You don't need to be extrasensory, have the option to see the soul, or know where it is explicitly to utilize this procedure.

Typically, when an individual's body passes on, the soul goes up to the light to be mended and favored. Nonetheless, in certain conditions, a soul will wind up confounded and not go to the light immediately. The element may stay near the earth plane and abide by well-known individuals or spots. The soul may end up influenced by lower wants and attempt to make issues for individuals. Generally, this includes taking individuals' vitality; making them feel frail. These spirits may cause disarray and different troubles including a weakness for the individuals they are in contact with. Some of the time they append themselves to an individual's air, making negative impacts, or they might be associated with a home, lodging, or other structure. On the off chance that you are working with a customer on a particular issue that doesn't appear to clear after a few sessions, the customer may have a soul waiting to be discharged. It's not important to tell the customer they have a soul except if you feel they will have the option to acknowledge this thought. In the event that you don't feel it insightful to tell the customer, essentially disclose to them you're going to utilize a propelled recuperating procedure.

The working suspicion with this strategy is that the soul is befuddled here and there and that is the motivation behind why they are causing issues. The soul should be recuperated so it can go to the light. This procedure isn't a trial of wills where you attempt to drive the soul out; it is a healing or mending procedure. Likewise, you won't utilize any of your own vitality in this procedure; an illuminated being will do the soul discharge process for you and that is the reason it is sheltered. This procedure can be utilized to discharge spirits from individuals and furthermore from areas; for example, from a home or fabricating or a territory.

Chapter 5: What Are the Other Applications Of Reiki?

Treating and Practicing Reiki On Other People

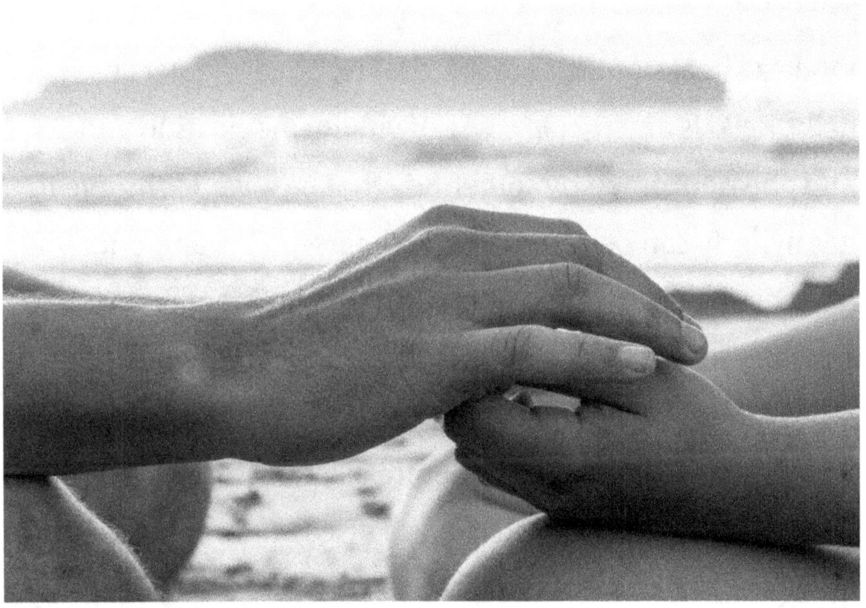

You can learn Reiki to give you a pragmatic method to take your wellbeing and prosperity into your very own hands. By figuring out how to move vitality and influence vigorous frameworks, you'll have the option to utilize that learning to improve your very own wellbeing and the soundness of your friends and family.

It's imperative to keep up a functioning nearness of healers in each network, and to learn Reiki is to get together with other characteristic healers around the globe to help make the world a more beneficial, progressively positive spot to live while simultaneously straightforwardly recuperating your prompt companions, family, and neighbors.

While all healers influence life vitality, not all healers use Reiki. Reiki is a particular type of vitality medication and must be performed by somebody that has been sensitive to it. Anybody can be receptive to rehearse Reiki, and once you have been adjusted you hold the endowment of Reiki for an amazing remainder.

Reiki is a piece of the Eastern enthusiastic restorative custom and is notwithstanding starting to discover a spot in western emergency clinics. Attendants and volunteers are accepting preparing and attunement, and in certain states, Reiki preparing fits the bill for nursing proceeding with training credits. Reiki is polished in networks far and wide, by regular individuals and by medicinal experts both in the option and conventional mending universes.

You can learn Reiki face-to-face through a class, or online through remote coursework. Regardless of whether instructed face to face or through a separation learning class, the advantages of Reiki training and attunement are the equivalent. The principle distinction is cost. In-person classes will, in general, be progressively costly, and frequently don't give much in the method for course materials for later reference.

Not every person who practices Reiki needs to utilize their preparation as a way to bring home the bacon. Be that as it may, filling in as a healer can be a wonderful profession. As a Reiki expert, you can invest heavily in your work and have any kind of effect on your customers' personal satisfaction.

In the event that you are pondering setting up a Reiki practice, consider the accompanying tips before beginning. It is best not to bounce in feet first setting up a Reiki practice until you have an unmistakable comprehension of your association with the activities of Reiki. Start encountering Reiki on an individual level through self-medication and treating relatives and companions.

Encountering all the inward functions of this delicate, complex recuperating craftsmanship requires some serious energy.

Reiki cleans up blockages and uneven characters step by step. Permit Reiki to enable you to get your very own life in parity before assuming the errand of helping other people.

You have the paper confirmation demonstrating that you have finished your Reiki preparing and are currently qualified as a Reiki specialist. Congrats! Lamentably, this bit of paper may be good for nothing with regards to legitimately offering proficient administrations in your general vicinity. Some U.S. states require a permit to rehearse characteristic wellbeing treatments. What's more, in light of the fact that Reiki is profound recuperating workmanship, in certain states, you might be required to end up guaranteed as an appointed clergyman.

Calling your nearby city corridor is a decent method to start your reality discovering mission; request to address somebody who can give you data about business licenses. A few regions additionally have this data on their sites; however, it may not be anything but difficult to discover. Consider acquiring risk protection for your insurance against potential claims.
You may likewise need to have customers sign a discharge

expressing that they have been educated that Reiki is definitely not a substitute for therapeutic consideration. Here is an example discharge you can adjust:

Vitality Work Consent and Release Statement:

I, the undersigned, comprehend that the Reiki session given includes a characteristic hands-on technique for vitality adjusting with the end goal of torment the board, stress decrease, and unwinding. We see plainly that these medications are not expected as a substitute for medicinal or mental consideration.

I comprehend that Reiki specialists don't analyze conditions, nor do they recommend meds, nor meddle with the treatment of an authorized restorative expert. It is suggested that I look for an authorized human service proficient for any physical or mental illness I have.

I comprehend that the specialist will place hands on me during the Reiki session.

Customer Name (Signature)

Reiki sessions are being offered in medical clinics, nursing homes, torment the executive's centers, spas, and locally established organizations. The advantage of working in a medical clinic, center, spa, or somewhere else is that arrangement appointments and protection guarantee filings are normally dealt with for you.

Most medical coverages don't repay for Reiki medicines; however, a couple does. Medicare in some cases pays for Reiki medicines if the sessions are endorsed for agony the executives.

Rehearsing from a locally situated office is a fantasy worked out as expected for some experts, yet this comfort accompanies issues to consider. Do you have a room or territory inside your home, separate from your ordinary living quarters that could be devoted to recuperating? Does the private zone you are living in permit locally established organizations? Furthermore, there is additionally the wellbeing issue of welcoming outsiders into your own living space to consider.

You will need to put resources into a solid back rub table for your training if the space you'll be rehearsing in doesn't have one. On the off chance that you offer to go so as to make home visits or give medicines in lodgings, a versatile back rub table will be fundamental. Here is an agenda of hardware and supplies for your Reiki practice:

- Back rub table

- Table frill

- Swivel seat with rollers

- Naturally cleaned materials

- Covers

- Cushions

- Tissues

- Filtered water

Informal exchange is a decent method to begin filling in as a Reiki professional. Tell your companions and relatives that you're open for business. Have business cards printed up and disseminate them uninhibitedly at neighborhood notice sheets at libraries, junior colleges, regular nourishment markets, and so on. Offer basic workshops and Reiki offers to instruct your locale about Reiki.

In the cutting-edge period, informal likewise means having a nearness via web-based networking media. Setting up a Facebook page for your training is free and just takes a couple of minutes. In a perfect world, you'll have your own site that rundowns your area and contact data, however in the event that that is distant, a Facebook page is a decent begin to attract new customers. Facebook likewise has devices that enable private ventures to contact a focused on a group of spectators (costs will shift).

Research what other Reiki specialists are charging in your general vicinity for their administrations. You will need to be focused, yet don't undermine yourself.
Do a money-saving advantage examination and expertise much you have to acquire—regardless of whether it's every hour, per quiet or per treatment—to cover your costs and have some cash left finished.
 In the event that you organize to treat customers outside of your home, odds are you will either pay a fixed rate for a

rental space or offer a level of your session expenses with your host business. Keep great records of the cash you are procuring. Filling in as a self-employed entity includes being educated regarding your personal assessment and independent work commitments.

Hand Positioning for Treating Other People

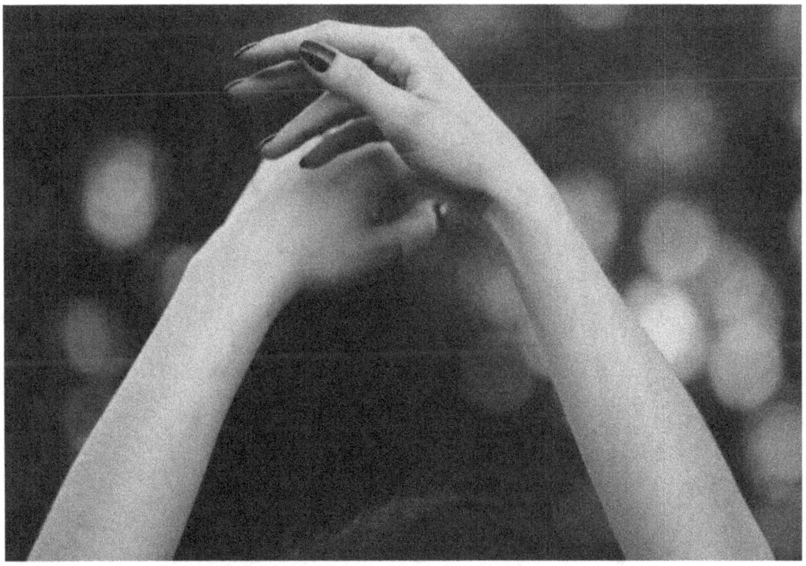

One note about body security; ordinarily the professional must place their hands exceptionally close (or on) body parts most consider to be private (genitalia). Since Reiki treats the whole body, it's ideal to not let such body parts alone for treatment. A few people genuinely need recuperating in their genitalia or other private body parts. Simultaneously there are matters of security to ensure, and the danger of maltreatment by the specialist. Fare thee well and do your work in an expert way.

Every specialist has their own specific manner to deal with this. It's great to advise the customer and ask consent before the session so that there are no curveballs. There are several different ways to work in these regions without straightforwardly reaching the customer's body and without bargaining the recuperating session. First is for the customer to put their very own hands on their body, at that point the professional places their hands over the customers' hands. The professional should "shaft" the vitality through the customers' hands. Another alternative is for the professional to hold their hands over those regions, with no contacting, and bar the vitality from a slight separation. Ultimately the separation recuperating images can be utilized.

Expert solace is very significant while rehearsing Reiki. A full treatment can without much of a stretch keep going for an hour and if the patient is lying on the floor by what method can the professional stay agreeable slouch over for that long? Better is for the patient to be situated in a seat that gives the specialist simple access to their entire body. Back rub tables are generally excellent for Reiki since they can be balanced, are agreeable, and enables the patient to loosen up more completely. A few organizations make tables implied explicitly for Reiki, which enables a move around the seat to go underneath the table.

In Reiki, there are essential customary and key hand positions instructed in Reiki confirmation courses that are utilized to advance vitality parity and help with mending to different territories of the body. Contingent upon your specific medical problem, additional time might be spent on one region than another during a Reiki treatment. This article features the essential Reiki hand positions, as a rule. A portion of the hand positions might be excluded and additionally, they may happen in an alternate request during a session. Minor departure from these positions may likewise be done, contingent upon your individual needs.

In case you're going in for your first treatment, these are the positions you can by and large hope to be utilized, as they are ordinary to most treatment sessions. Each position is intended to adjust the energies around there and evacuate stuck energies there so you can start to unwind, decrease pressure and enable space for your body to rest and mend and to work all the more ideally. On the off chance that you need specific consideration set on one zone, do tell your professional. Ordinarily, your expert will have the option to detect regions inside the hand places that need additional consideration you might not have even known required it.

During a Reiki session, a customer lays serenely on a back rub table or is now and then situated on a seat. There is no control of tissue as in back rub or bodywork that happens, yet only an exceptionally delicate hand weight. What's more, not normal for back rub treatment, you are in every case completely dressed during a Reiki session. The session is typically done peacefully with negligible talking, except if obviously, you wish to impart something to your expert, at that point, it is significant that you do so instantly during the session. Your Reiki specialist may play calm alleviating mood melodies or nature sounds.

In the event that you are awkward or could be progressively agreeable, for instance, if the music is diverting or in the event that you want to skirt a certain Reiki hand position, simply let your expert know previously or during your session.

Reiki is performed with either exceptionally delicate, static weight from the specialist's hands on conventional hand position territories, or with their hands drifting a couple of creeps over your body. Reiki works similarly too in either case so on the off chance that you want to not be contacted legitimately with any of the majority of the hand positions and lean toward the floating technique, it would be ideal if you impart that to your expert previously or during your session. Delicate or private territories are never contacted during a Reiki session. Regardless of whether you have a medical problem in a delicate or private zone, it is against a Reiki Professional Practitioner's Code of Ethics to physically contact private or touchy territories. Your Reiki Practitioner needs you to have the most unwinding and agreeable experience as would be prudent while you appreciate this ageless technique for Japanese vitality work for pressure decrease, unwinding, and health.

Here are probably the most widely recognized general hand places that you may understand during your Reiki session:

Position A: Palms are set softly on your temple as well as the expert's hands may delicately cup your eyes.

Position B: The specialist may soothingly put their hands around along the edges of your sanctuaries and face.

Position C: Your head might be supported in the specialist's hands as their hands lay on the table.

Position D: Your facial structure or throat region may delicately be offered Reiki.

Position E: The expert's privilege or left hand may float or be set close to your neck or over your collarbones, while their other hand will drift or be set over your heart chakra.

Position F: Hands might be set tenderly on your upper belly.

Position G: The specialist may put their hands on your sun-based plexus region or mid-belly

Position H: The professional may put their hands on your mid-lower mid-region, a couple of creeps underneath your navel.

Position I: Optionally a professional may offer Reiki to your knees or potentially to your lower legs or feet. These are discretionary positions if the specialist feels they may profit you. On the other hand, they may essentially proceed onward to hand positions on your back.

Position J: The specialist may ask for, on the off chance that you are on a back rub table, that you rest tenderly to the other side. The professional's hands are tenderly set on your shoulder bone zone and rest there.

Position K: Hands are descended to a situation under you should cutting edges or center back.

Position L: The professional moves their hands to apply delicate weight in a hand position at your lower back.

When the essential positions and additionally varieties have all been secured and stuck energies expelled or adjusted, the professional may move their hands over your body in a general movement to scrub your vitality field of any extra vitality flotsam and jetsam, leaving you scrubbed, feeling better, and well on your approach to upgraded prosperity.

A short time later, if it's not too much trouble make certain to drink a lot of water for 24 hours after your session and to take some time, even only two or three minutes, to delight in the serenity and peacefulness after your session. Attempt to permit 10 or 15 minutes at some point after your session or maybe later in the prior night bed to get thankfulness from your higher self for thinking about your body, brain, and soul and to make the most of your expanded condition of wellbeing and harmony.

When conducting a Reiki treatment, there are twelve key positions for the hands.

Face: The hands are placed of the face of the recipient. The palms gently recognize the sanctuary thus gently estimating the eyes with the fingers. Be mindful of the recipient' s airways by not blocking the nostrils' pathways.

Crown and Top of the Head: With your internal wrists reaching fold your hands over the recipient's head, empowering your fingertips to contact the ears.

Back of the Head: Hands should be tucked beneath the recipient' s head. A pleasant outline needs to be set out for the head. Then, the back of the hands is used to loosen up and the on the table or a pad if available.

Jaw and Jawline: The recipient's face is surrounded by the hands. The tips of your fingers are empowered to contact beneath the face and enhance the effect purposes of hands close to or gently covering the ears.

Neck Collarbone and Heart: Daintily wrap the right hand on the neck of the recipient. Or on the other hand if the recipient is cumbersome, empower your hand to coast to some degree over the neck. Your left arm should be stretched going further down to set the hand over the center of the heart.

Ribs and Rib Cage: On the upper section of the ribs, place hands directly beneath the chest. Keep in mind that touch of private areas is not appropriate during treatment of others.

Mid-area: Hands are placed on the stomach, or the area known as the "solar plexus", that is, over the belly button of the recipient.

Pelvic Bones: Your hands should be placed on each of your pelvic bones.

Shoulder Bones: The recipient should be helped to change positions, moving from laying down on the back to laying down on the stomach.

The " Ninth" position: Hands should be set upon the shoulder blades. In this location, the place enthusiastic loads are consistently taken care of; thus, there is a need for your palms to remain in this form for a segment of time for the other hand circumstances to help unstick stuck energies.

Midback: Set the hands upon the inside area of the back.

Lower Back: As one continues down the back of the body, spot hands on the lower back section of the recipient.

Sacrum: At the end of the session, the recipient is brushed by the expert with a sweep of the hand to gather any enthusiastic remains that have been lifted from the physical body as a result of the treatment. Greater benefit can be achieved by taking peaceful interest in positive energies thereby clearing about negative ones. Then, negative energies are removed and set back out into the universe.

All About Scanning Aura

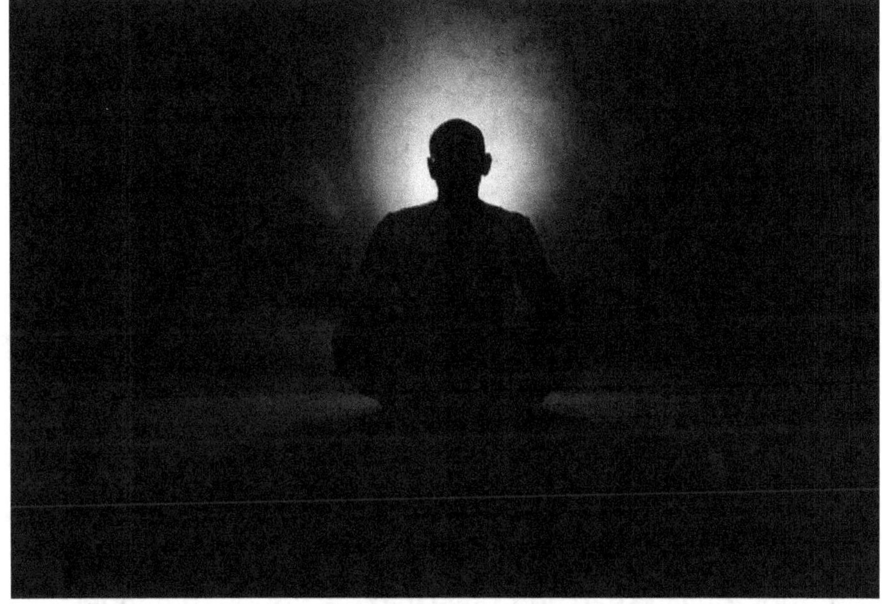

Emanation, also known as an Aura, is the bio-electric field that encompasses we all. It is extremely useful to figure out how to check the Aura in light of the fact that the vast majority of the sicknesses and issues begin and have their underlying foundations in our Aura. Each living thing on the earth transmits a field of vitality, which is called an atmosphere of vitality checking. In people, there are seven primary focuses in the body that produce the vitality or the quality, and these vitality focuses are called Chakras. These vitality fields can be looked over a long separation and afterward translated in the examination. The investigation gives an ideal assessment of the material and otherworldly status of a person.

Since the early Vedic period, Indian sages have related air (Tej or Abha Mandal) with perfect and profound forces. The iridescent corona around the paintings of divine beings and holy people are simply unmistakable development of the quality, the vitality handle that interpenetrates, express and pervade both our gross and inconspicuous substances.

Indeed, even present-day researchers have done significant looks into about Aura. Kirlean photography has achieved a significant high status. With the assistance of Kirlian photography, researchers have had the option to ponder, watch, and take pictures of little bioplasmic articles like bioplasmic fingers, leaves, and so forth.

When we recuperate the Aura, we are destroying the reason as well as get the chance to mend issues in their underlying stages before they get an opportunity to appear in our physical body and reality.

An extra advantage of mending the Aura before treatment is that the individual will be increasingly open in tolerating the

Reiki and will enable it to stream all the more effectively to a zone that necessities recuperating the most. When we are receptive to Reiki, our palm chakras open up which increase their affectability in identifying energies.

What establishes an Aura? The air is halfway made from EM (electromagnetic) radiation, spreading over from microwave, infrared (IR) to UV light.

Low recurrence microwave and infrared piece of the range (body heat) are identified with the low degrees of the working of our body (DNA structure, digestion, dissemination and so on.) while high recurrence (UV part) related with our cognizant movement; for example, thinking, innovativeness, expectations, comical inclination and feelings.

The arrangement, layers, shape, profundity, and multi-shades of the Aura make it so noticeable, spiritualist and awesome that it goes to valuable for an examination of the people. Every Aura contains seven layers. These are described below:

Etheric layer: It delineates the physical condition. It shapes a splendid hover around a solid individual, while it is pale appearance around a weak individual.

Enthusiastic layer: Depicts the status of feelings.

Mental layer: It mirrors the inward vitality of an individual and shows self-control.

Astral layer: The focal astral layer is associated with heart, gives a connection between body, psyche and soul and interfaces the person with other living creatures known to mankind. It is huge and splendid in the individuals who worth associations with others.

Etheric layer: The vitality field of correspondence and inventive articulation. Blockage, dark brown spots/mists or haziness in this layer show the sentiment of confinement.

Divine layer: Represents the visual faculties. It additionally mirrors a person's standpoint about the remainder of the world.

Ketheric layer: Linked with self-assurance and basic leadership capacity. When it is sparkling brilliantly, it shows a mind unafraid of decisions and analysis by others.

It is accepted that human quality has seven noteworthy levels. The physical and etheric levels reach out around six crawls to a foot from the physical body. The imaginal and passionate auric levels stretch out around two feet from the body, joining the physical and etheric levels. The psychological, prototype, and profound airs degree around three feet from the body and join different levels.

The vitality checking enables us to see the examination of the vital elements that impact the body-mind work. A CESS (Computerized Energy Scanning System) is utilized to follow out different positive and negative vibrations. This vibration mirrors the inward condition of vitality; for example, Mental, enthusiastic, and intuitive energies.

The auric example rather gives a substantially more complete picture as respects reasonable condition of occurring. It shows upon relationship concordance, achievement in work, obstacles and snags to be wary upon, general physical and enthusiastic wellbeing. The examination is extremely noteworthy in light of the fact that not an individual find out about the pluses and minuses, yet in addition, have a remedial arrangement. On the off chance that and where required, quality and chakra purging is additionally exhorted.

Figuring out how to body examine in Reiki is generally instructed in Level II of the Reiki preparing. This body checking is an opening of the third eye chakra so as to see energies that are needing being unblocked from the body. On the off chance that you are rehearsing Reiki, there are a few distinct procedures that you can utilize when figuring out how to body filter.

The main thing that one will figure out how to do with body filtering is the means by which to discover certain emanations. These are vitality forms that are situated all through a people body. When one needs recuperating, they may find that there is a piece of an emanation that is an opening or a dull spot in the body.

When one is beginning, they can discover these energies by putting somebody before a white divider and change the manner by which you take a gander at them. When you are polished at this, you will have the option to detect the energies simpler. There are likewise a few machines that are presently ready to indicate someone's atmosphere.

Hand Scanning

Many will likewise practice body looking over the utilization of their hands. You can clear your hands over your very own or someone's body. After some time, you will figure out how to perceive where the vitality is and where it is blocked. Some of the time, the energies will differentiate so much that you will have the option to discover regions on the body that convey an unexpected temperature in comparison to the remainder of the body. These temperature contrasts show a square of vitality.

Pendulums are another normal strategy for body examining. You can move a pendulum here and there a body. It will indicate zones where the vitality is off by not keeping a similar beat all through the body. The pendulum should move in various ways between the diverse chakras. At the point when the pendulum doesn't move in a roundabout movement, yet vertically rather, it demonstrates that there is an issue with the vitality around there.

Body Energy

Body filtering will make you have the option to see

distinctive vitality streams by the adjustments in vitality from either your own body or from another person. Warmth and coolness is frequently detected change in energies.

There are additionally once in a while events of shivering, electric stuns, heartbeats, or pulling sensations. These vitality changes will demonstrate to you where the body's energies are off and will demonstrate to you what to do so as to change the vitality stream with all-inclusive vitality.

When you discover the issue spots with vitality stream, you can draw nearer to that territory. From here, you will have the option to pull in the all-inclusive energies and use them to evacuate the blockage. After you have wrapped up this blockage, you can re-check the territory where there were issues so as to ensure that it is offset with the remainder of the vitality.

By realizing how to body filter, one can without much of a stretch become a piece of the Reiki recuperating process and have the option to mend others. Examining a body is one of the significant systems that are utilized with Reiki. While there are no set approaches to discover vitality hinders, every one of them will help to rebalance and take into consideration the vitality stream to travel through one's body.

The Process:

Actuate and stimulate the chakras in your palms utilizing Cho Ku Rei image.

Shield and ground yourself utilizing certifications or through perception.

Start by setting your non-predominant hand around 10 inches from the customers Crown Chakra. Move your attention to your palms and notice how the vitality feels.

Draw your hand nearer to the customer at around 5 inches. Keep this separation steady and begin to move your palm from the customers Crown Chakra to the bottoms of his feet.

Do this gradually monitoring every one of the impressions that you experience as you move the hands through the Aura.

You will feel sensations like pushing, pulling, changes in

temperature, shivering, stuns, unevenness, obstruction and so on to give some examples.

As you practice an ever-increasing number of these sensations will turn out to be anything but difficult to identify and they will turn out to be progressively noticeable and clear.

When you can recognize the zone that requirements recuperating check if the territory is exhausted of vitality or is there a blockage? Consumption feels like an empty and blockages feel like bulges.

Move your hand here and there on that region until you discover the stature where you feel the most twisting. This could be a few feet from the part or very close contingent upon the kind of issue.

When you locate the correct stature, cup both your hands and spot it on the influenced region and ask Reiki to move through you and do the recuperating. Keep on recuperating the influenced territory until the Reiki stops to stream.

Check for comparable diseases in the air and apply a similar technique.

Body filtering is a significant piece of most Reiki mending sessions. Body filtering is an instinctive strategy for recognizing zones of the body needing mending.

Reiki experts, who acknowledge the significance of chakras in mending, talk about opening the "third eye" so as to see energies that should be unblocked. The thought is that issues inside the body will appear inside the individual's atmospheres.

For instance, the disease may air with a gap in it or a surprising dim spot. Figuring out how to see airs and unsettling influences in emanations takes practice. On the off chance that atmospheres are incorporated as a feature of your Reiki preparing, you will be given activities that help you figure out how to see the unobtrusive emanations encompassing an individual.

Clairvoyant Scanning

Clairvoyant Scanning is a strategy that includes mystically examining the body, organs; Aura and Energy points

(Chakras).

A sweep is a natural procedure of finding issues or distress that would then be able to be tended to, whenever required by a medicinal expert. Mystic filtering is certifiably not a substitute for authorized medicinal consideration and doesn't replace x-beams or MRI's that might be requested by your doctor. Mystic Scanning can help distinguish territories where physical issues may show whenever left untreated.

It is an astounding procedure to use with people; for example, the incapacitated, the youthful, or the older who may somehow not have the option to convey distress or other wellbeing concerns. It is a brilliant chance to get understanding into your very own wellbeing or to discover how a friend or family member is feeling who probably won't have the option to convey something else. Body sweeps should be possible on any individual or creature around the globe. All the data that is gotten will be given to the endless supply of the sweep. Anyway, there is no assurance that Psychic Scanning is 100% precise.

Clairvoyant Healing

A clairvoyant healer is an individual who can channel his mystic vitality towards easing a condition or mending the body in a comprehensive manner. The mystic healer may utilize instinctive, extrasensory or clairvoyant abilities to detect and recuperate a physical affliction. There are additionally clairvoyant diagnosticians or medicinal natural that can touch base at an analysis of what's going on with an individual's body without utilizing any restorative devices like x-beams or sweeps.

Some recuperating modalities that perhaps utilized by clairvoyant healers are Reiki, pranic mending procedures, guided symbolism, inventive representation, assertions in a mix with herbs, back rub, fragrance-based treatment and dietary eating routine changes.

Body filtering can be utilized toward the start, during, and toward the finish of a Reiki mending session. When it is done before a Reiki recuperating session, examines furnish healers with development data on where to think their endeavors. Utilized during a mending session, examines help healers realize when to respite to channel Reiki and when to proceed onward.

 Toward the finish of a session, a re-output of the body

guarantees that the progression of vitality through the body has been improved and is currently adjusted.

Chapter 6: Other Reiki Exercises and Healing Materials

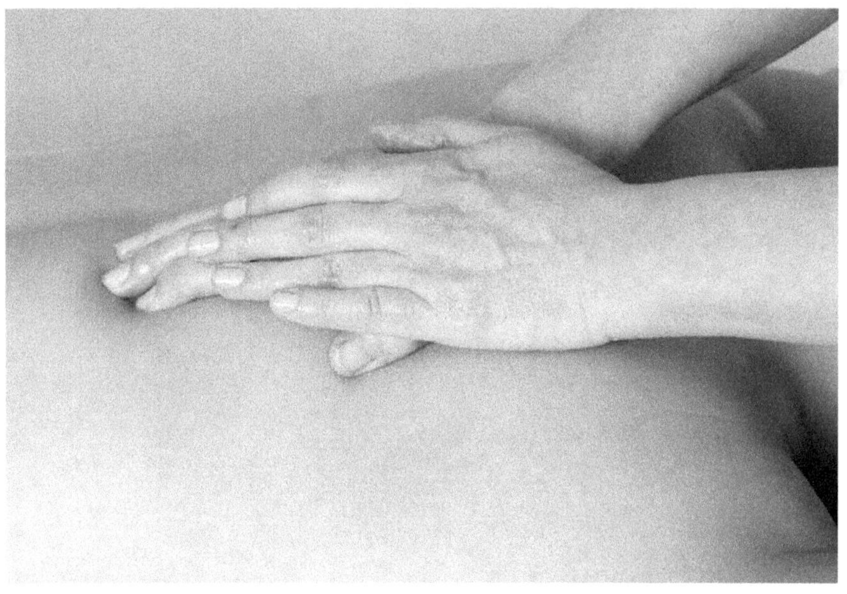

Reiki has been known to be used as an elective form of treatment as a part of essentialness recovery. It gained popularity in the late 1800s in Japan and it is said to incorporate the generalities of the essentialness straight from the palms of the expert to the recipient.

Experts have utilized Essentialness repairing under several structures for a great deal of time. Supporters state that it is effective within the essentialness areas of the body.

There is a lot of talk regarding Reiki nowadays due to the fact that it does not always get consistent results through the use of its common techniques. In any event, recipients of Reiki claim that it is effective thereby boosting its reputation. A Google search will reveal over 68 million results.

Recent research conducted highlights the fact that over 1.2 million adults sought some form of Reiki therapy in the United States at least once in the last year. There are over 60 recognized centers in the United States which offer some kind of Reiki therapy to their patients.

"Reiki" implies "hidden air, superb sign." The name " Reiki" is derived from the Japanese terms " rei" which means " general" and " ki" which means " essentialness of life" . As such, Reiki implies a " general essentialness of life" as a result of touching the individual with the healing energy of the universe.

Consequently, this healing touch surrounds the body in such a way that the energy stimulates the natural healing mechanisms of the body.

As shown by experts, essentialness may stall inside the physical body in cases where there has been some type of harm or perhaps emotional distress. Over time, these episodes may lead to the rise of a disorder.

Imperativeness solution intends to help the movement of essentialness and clear upsets thusly to needle treatment or weight point knead. Improving the movement of imperativeness around the body, as said by specialists, can enable loosening up, decline torment, speed recovering, and reduce distinctive reactions of the disease.

Reiki has been around for an enormous number of years. The case of Mikao Usui is a clear example of how Reiki can be used to heal especially when considering that he trained over 2,000 people in this art over the course of his lifetime.

The art of Reiki then made its way into the United Sates, through Hawaii, in the 1940s. Later on, it spread into Europe in the 1980s. Reiki was easily identifiable as the healing action of placing one's hands over the recipient.

Yet, what actually goes on during a Reiki intervention?

The best way to practice Reiki is in a quite and peaceful environment. Nevertheless, it can continue anywhere, at any time. The recipient is asked to sit in a comfortable position, or perhaps lie on a table, while begin totally clothed. Music could be used to enhance the mood depending on the recipient' s preference. Next, the expert' s hands are gently placed over the areas corresponding to the head, limbs, and the core by using a series of hand positions for some place in the scope of 2 and 5 minutes. The hands can be set in excess of 20 remarkable zones of the body.

In case there is explicit harm, for instance, the damaged part should be the main focus of the hands. This should be done while the expert' s hands are softly placed on top of the body. At this point, the hands of the expert might show signs of warmth and slight trembling. Each of the positions carried out by the hands must be held until the expert can see that the essentialness has ceased to spill.

At the moment when the giver of the energy feels that the essentialness in their grip has begun to calm down, they will then release their hands and place them on top of a substitute area of the recipient' s body.

How to Use Reiki When Healing Ailments?

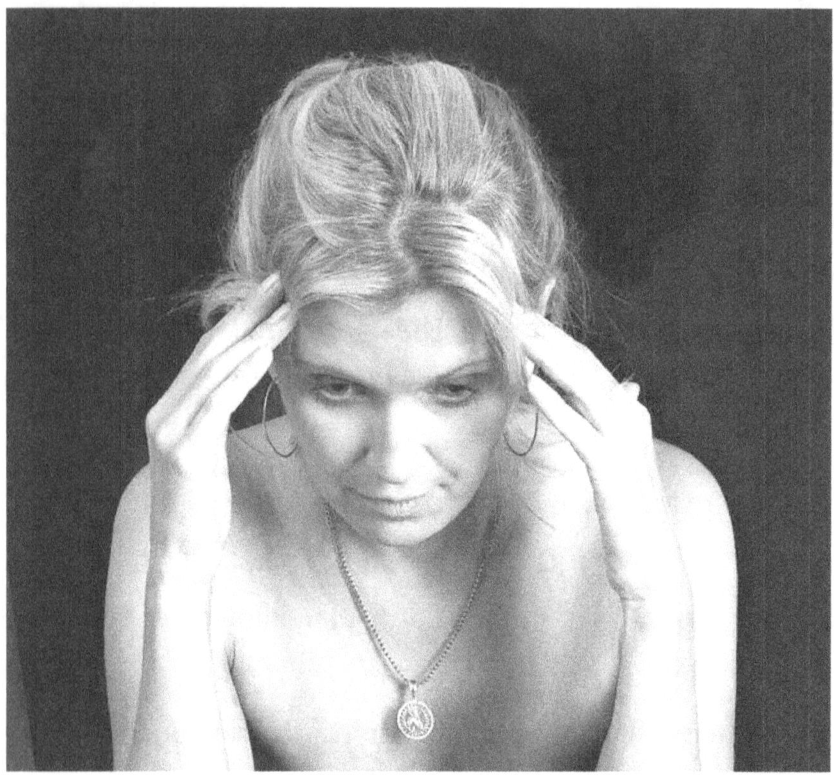

As indicated by experts, the mending impacts are interceded by diverting the general vitality Which received the name of " qi" , articulated "chi." The word for this term in India is "prana." It is a similar vitality associated with judo work out. It is the existence of power vitality that some accept encompasses we all.

This vitality is said to pervade the body. Reiki specialists bring up that, while this vitality isn't quantifiable by present-day logical strategies, it tends to be felt by numerous who check out it.

Reiki is affirmed to help to unwind, aid the body's regular recuperating forms, and create enthusiastic, mental, and otherworldly prosperity.

It is additionally said to incite profound unwinding, help individuals adapt to troubles, diminish enthusiastic pressure, and improve in general prosperity.

Individuals who get Reiki portray it as "strongly unwinding."

Here are some examples of health conditions which Reiki has been known to help sufferers manage:

-Malignancy

-Coronary illness

-Uneasiness

-Sorrow

-Incessant torment

-Barrenness

-Neurodegenerative issue

-Chemical imbalance

-Crohn's sickness

-Weariness disorders

According to research conducted by University of Minnesota, individuals who have experienced a Reiki intervention have stated that:

"I feel invigorated and appear to think all the more unmistakably."

"I think I nodded off."

"I can't accept how hot your hands got!"

"I feel looser than even after a back rub."

"My cerebral pain is no more."

Malignancy sufferers that undergo Reiki therapy state they notice improvement following a session. This may be in light of the fact that it makes them loosen up. Another clarification, as demonstrated by Cancer Research U.K. could be that Reiki contributes vitality with them and gets in touch with them. This soothingly influences recipients that might become overwhelmed by the nature of traditional treatment in addition to the stress, anxiety and fear that comes along with it.

Recipients indicate varying experiences. Some recipients have indicated that the expert's hands feel warm, while others manifest that they have felt a cooling sensation in the form of waves. Some of the most notable accounts show that feelings of stress and anxiety quickly begin to dissipate.

No prior planning, guidance, or training is needed to get started with Reiki therapy. There is no need for any type of "attunement process", either. It has been said that Reiki is a type of "notable supernatural condition" in which the expert is believed to have attuned their essentialness to a point in which the recovery techniques used are effective on the recipient.

While training for Reiki differs somewhat, most students received training on:

The energies that surround the physical vessel.

The most effective method of working with healing energies.

The morals applied when dealing with recipients.

The attunement process for a healing session may include fasting for a period of 2 to 3 days, meditation, focus on nature and the dissipation of negative emotions.

There exist three degrees of mastery. Those individuals who attain the "Ace" level can demonstrate their mastery to others by becoming ready to help those who seek their aid. Nevertheless, as Reiki gains more and more popularity, some questions linger.

Reiki cases to empower unwinding, diminish torment, speed mending, and improve a few indications; however, few research discoveries bolster particular medical advantages. It has been scrutinized for professing to recuperate illnesses without logical proof. Some have portrayed its cases as fake.

Pundits state that it goes against our present comprehension of the laws of nature. Supporters react that the advantages of prosperity and decreased pressure are genuine yet difficult to quantify with a logical report.

Researchers note that top-notch examination into its viability is deficient. No investigation has yet demonstrated that it is any more successful than a fake treatment, as experts state.

A 2008 study concluded that there was no conclusive evidence to support the effectiveness of Reiki as a means of treatment for any of the conditions it claims to have healed. This has led to Reiki' s effectiveness being called into question.

A 2015 study focused on Reiki and its contributions to the treatment of emotional conditions such as anxiety. The researchers concluded that they were "lacking the proof to state whether Reiki is valuable for individuals more than 16 years old with uneasiness or despondency or both." Unfortunately, the research that has been conducted on the subject has been subpar and has not met scientific standards such as using control groups or patient surveys.

Research conducted by BMC Nephrology on the use of Reiki in dialysis patients, has shown that such patients have been benefitted by "mending contact". The study looked into the treatment offered by volunteers in which recipients also indicated a reduction in negative feelings associated to their condition and a sense of "accomplishing something" as patients reported some degree of relief.

Recently, Annie Harrington of the UK Reiki Federation told MNT that there has been "enormous report recording much of the preliminary research" done into Reiki. As such, it would appear that discoveries have been made with regard to Reiki's effectiveness. In addition, the UK's Complementary and Natural Healthcare Council (CNHC) has been looking into supporting Reiki enter mainstream treatment options.

That being said, it is worth nothing that Reiki centers offering such healing services to the general public are now asked to become compliant with local laws by adding disclaimers to their publicity indicating that Reiki is not an official course of treatment. Moreover, it is not used to test, diagnose or heal and medical conditions. Furthermore, the Advertising Standards Agency (ASA) in the UK has denied claims supporting Reiki as a means of healing various medical conditions.

Research conducted by Physics Procedia under the direction of Judy Kosovich has provided a " new look" at the guidelines for vitality medication. In short, current legislation and oversight into the medical profession do have people' s security in mind, it is also known that there still much which is unknown about the human body by mainstream science.

As such, this has called Reiki' s safety into question. The US National Center for Complementary and Integrative Health (NCCIH) has expressed opinions about Reiki by stating that it " has not been unmistakably demonstrated to be valuable for any wellbeing related reason" . And while this opinion does not express support for the therapeutics of Reiki, it does not claim that Reiki has any negative effects, either.

The principle concern gives off an impression of being that individuals with genuine medical problems may decide on Reiki and other reciprocal treatments rather than thoroughly tried present-day medication. Nonetheless, utilizing it nearby different medications is probably not going to be dangerous.

In fact, contact alone, regardless of whether with or without "all-inclusive vitality," seems to have a scope of advantages, from structure trust to upgrading generally speaking prosperity.

Kosovich brings up that costly ordinary medications that are right now accessible regularly have genuine antagonistic impacts and could possibly work. Numerous individuals, subsequently, might want the opportunity to pick an option.

Reiki: Its Role in Treating Autoimmune Diseases

Immune system maladies can influence individuals of all ages or foundation. At the point when these maladies build-up, the manifestations run from gentle to crippling, frequently lessening the personal satisfaction for the sufferer. Contingent upon the infection, various medicines may exist. Be that as it may, paying little mind to the idea of the immune system condition, people enduring with these maladies may likewise profit by an elective treatment known as "Reiki."

Understanding Autoimmune Diseases

Immune system infections happen when the safe framework glitches. The motivation behind the insusceptible framework is to shield the body from trespassers that might be destructive; for example, infections and microscopic organisms. Nonetheless, now and again, the insusceptible framework experiences difficulty perceiving the contrast between outside materials and the body's very own tissues. At the point when this happens, the invulnerable framework may erroneously assault the body's very own tissues, which prompts the advancement of immune system illnesses. Instances of normal immune system illnesses incorporate celiac malady, Grave's sickness, Type I diabetes, different sclerosis, incendiary entrail ailment, and rheumatoid joint inflammation. Much of the time, these ailments must be dealt with progressing therapeutic medications.

Advantages of Reiki for Patients with Autoimmune Disease

Patients with immune system ailments may profit by Reiki in various ways. A portion of these potential advantages may include:

Help with Pain

For some, immune system illnesses, torment is one of the most vexatious side effects. Patients with rheumatoid joint pain, incendiary gut malady or numerous scleroses, for instance, all arrangement with agony all the time. Numerous patients who have experienced Reiki medicines report feeling less torment because of the sessions. Hence, individuals who have immune system sicknesses may profit by fewer torment sensations in the event that they take an interest in Reiki treatment normally.

Better Sense of Physical and Emotional Balance

Numerous Reiki customers report feeling progressively adjusted due to their sessions, both physically and inwardly. This feeling of parity makes it simpler for individuals to manage their incessant sickness, and it improves their general personal satisfaction.

Less Anxiety as well as Depression

Both uneasiness and despondency are basic issues among individuals doing combating a lifetime immune system malady. Since there could possibly be a solution for these ailments, patients frequently feel sad. What's more, since side effects go back and forth, numerous patients likewise feel on edge about how their conditions will advance starting with one day then onto the next. Sadly, this state of mind aggravations just exacerbates the patients' side effects. Research studies have demonstrated that standard Reiki sessions may lessen sentiments of nervousness and improve the state of mind of customers. Not exclusively would this be able to improve the person's general condition, yet it might likewise make the person in question progressively agreeable with other recommended medicinal medications.

More advantageous Immune Function

Research with respect to Reiki's impact on insusceptible capacity is deficient. In any case, numerous patients with immune system illnesses report a decrease in side effects in the wake of experiencing Reiki medicines. Besides, there is no proof that Reiki is unsafe to individuals with these conditions, so it is a generally safe decision for individuals searching for common treatment choices.

A few people with malignancy may utilize Reiki close by their treatment, as a correlative treatment. Reiki experts state that it can: help you to feel profoundly loosened up assistance you adapt to troublesome circumstances diminish enthusiastic pressure and strain help to improve generally prosperity Some individuals with malignant growth state they feel better in the wake of utilizing treatments; for example, Reiki. Studies demonstrate this is frequently in light of the fact that a specialist invests energy with the individual and contacts them. After the surge and worry of emergency clinics and treatment, it tends to be loosening up when somebody gives you consideration for an hour or more, in a quiet setting. Reiki is now and then utilized in palliative consideration, particularly in hospices. A few people say that Reiki has controlled symptoms of their disease medications; for example, agony, tension, and ailment. They likewise state that it encourages them to adapt better to their disease and its treatment. In any case, it's imperative to tolerate at the top of the priority list that while Reiki may assist you with coping with your side effects or reactions, it can't treat your malignant growth.

On your first visit, your Reiki specialist will get some information about your general wellbeing and therapeutic history. They will ask you for what good reason you might want to have Reiki and talk about your treatment plan with you. You don't need to get uncovered for treatment. You more often than not take your shoes and coat off and make them sit or rest. You can have your eyes open or shut. Your Reiki expert may diminish the lights or play alleviating music. They put their hands on, or a couple of crawls over your body. They move their hands over your body, typically beginning at your head and working down to your feet; however, may concentrate on specific zones of the body.

The point is to move and adjust the 'vitality' inside and around your body. What's more, to dispose of any vitality squares to empower mending and reinforce your vitality. You may feel a shivering sensation, a profound unwinding, or warmth or coolness all through your body. Or on the other hand, you probably won't feel anything by any means. Experts state this doesn't mean the treatment isn't working. A session, for the most part, keeps going between 20 minutes and 60 minutes. Numerous professionals state you will get the best outcomes from 3 sessions inside a genuinely short space of time.

At that point enjoy a reprieve before having more medicines. You may feel parched after a session. It can drink a lot of water and maintain a strategic distance from solid caffeine-based beverages; for example, espresso. You may feel profoundly loose and resting at home subsequently can enable you to get the full advantage of the treatment. Reiki professionals state that Reiki can be sent remotely, over a separation. So, you can be in your very own home having Reiki from an individual somewhere else. In the event that you don't feel great with anything, it's essential to talk about this with your expert.

Remember that Reiki sessions are not a substitute for standard therapeutic treatment. Be that as it may, numerous individuals experiencing immune system ailments have announced advantages when Reiki was added to their treatment routine.

Numerous individuals are rehearsing methods to improve their wellbeing; for example, contemplation, exercise, and improved eating regimen.

As this is done, more profound mindfulness regularly creates concerning the progression of unpretentious energies in and around the body and the association between these unobtrusive energies and one's wellbeing. This creating mindfulness approves the antiquated thought of 'life power vitality' as the reason for wellbeing and its need as the reason for ailment.The presence of 'life power vitality' and the need for it to stream uninhibitedly in and around one's body to keep up wellbeing has been considered and recognized by medicinal services professionals just as researchers.

Our body is made not just out of physical components; for example, muscles, bones, nerves, supply routes, organs, organs, and so forth.; it likewise has an unpretentious vitality framework through which 'life power vitality' streams. This inconspicuous vitality framework is made out of vitality 'bodies' which encompass our physical body and help us in preparing our musings and feelings. The vitality bodies have vitality focuses called chakras, which work to some degree like valves that permit life power to flow through the physical, mental, passionate and profound bodies. We likewise have vitality meridians and points.
These resemble waterways or streams, which convey our life power vitality all through our physical body, to feed us and

help with adjusting our body's frameworks and capacities.

Our physical body is alive on account of the 'existence power vitality' that is streaming however it. On the off chance that our 'life power' is low or blocked, we are bound to become ill, yet on the off chance that it is high and free streaming, we all the more effectively keep up wellbeing and sentiment of prosperity. One thing that disturbs and debilitates the progression of 'life power vitality' is pressure. Stress is regularly brought about by clashing musings and emotions that get held up in one's unpretentious vitality framework. These incorporate dread, stress, question, outrage, uneasiness, and so forth. Restorative research has established that ceaseless pressure can obstruct the body's normal capacity to fix, recover and ensure itself. The American Institute of Stress appraises that 75% - 95% of all visits to specialists are the aftereffects of response to push. The impacts of unreleased pressure extend from minor longs to significant wellbeing concerns; for example, coronary illness, stomach related issue, respiratory and skin issues.

Reiki is a method that guides the body in discharging pressure and strain by making profound unwinding. Along these lines, Reiki advances recuperating and wellbeing. The word Reiki is made of two Japanese words - Rei, which signifies "the Wisdom of God," or the Higher Power" and Ki, which signifies "life power vitality." So Reiki signifies 'profoundly guided life power vitality.' The Reiki arrangement of mending is a strategy for transmitting this unobtrusive vitality to yourself as well as other people through the hands into the human vitality framework. Reiki reestablishes vitality parity and imperativeness by diminishing the physical and passionate impacts of unreleased pressure. It delicately and adequately opens blocked meridians and chakras, and clears the vitality bodies, leaving one inclination loose and settled.

Reiki can:

-Quicken recuperating

-Help the body in purging poisons

-Equalization the progression of unpretentious vitality by discharging blockages

-Help the customer contact the "healer inside."

A treatment feels like warm, delicate daylight which courses through you, encompasses you and solaces you. Reiki treats the individual's body, feelings, psyche, and soul in general. Reiki is a basic, normal and safe technique for profound mending and personal growth that everybody can utilize.

Reiki is incredible, yet superbly delicate and sustaining. During a treatment, the customers remain completely dressed. Reiki is a compelling option or supplement to rub treatment.

Anybody can figure out how to take advantage of a boundless stock of 'life power vitality' to improve wellbeing and upgrade the personal satisfaction by learning Reiki, or by getting medications from a Reiki Practitioner or Master.

Mental, Emotional, And Spiritual Healing

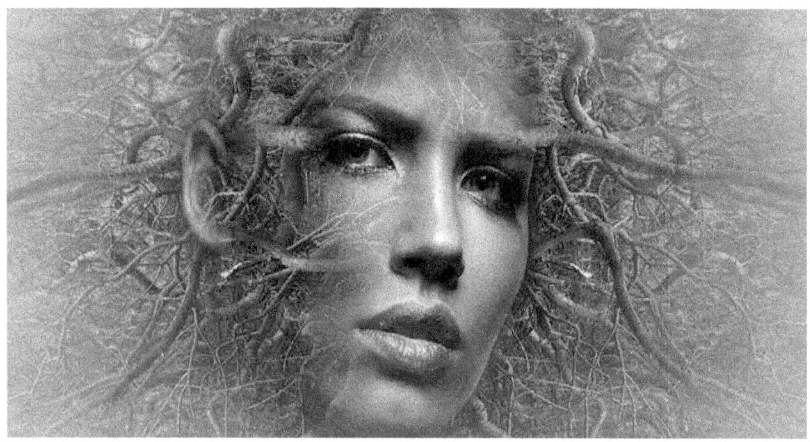

A commonplace Reiki session endures somewhere in the range of 20 and an hour and a half. At your first arrangement, you'll meet with your Reiki specialist. You'll have a short presentation or visit about the procedure and your desires or aims. Tell your expert about any manifestations you need to be tended to or if there are puts in the body on which you'd like them to center. Additionally, let the professional know whether you have any wounds or places that are touchy to contact.

You'll be told to rests on a treatment table or tangle. They will cover you with a cover. Typically delicate, loosening up music will play out of sight. Generally, there won't be any talking during the session; however, you can don't hesitate to fill your specialist in regarding whether there's something you have to feel increasingly great or to share what you're encountering.

The expert will move their hands around your body. They may contact you gently or have their hands simply over your body.

You may encounter sensations in the body; for example, warmth or shivering. A few people report seeing representations; for example, hues or pictures, or having recollections show up. Attempt to permit whatever emerges to go without appending a lot of importance to it. Your encounters may wind up further the more you proceed with Reiki.

Reiki is a Japanese vitality recuperating procedure. The prevailing type of Reiki rehearsed all through the present reality, otherwise called Usui Reiki, was made by Dr. Mikao Usui in the mid-twentieth century.

It's a correlative or elective wellbeing methodology. Reiki doesn't legitimately fix maladies or diseases. Rather, it's utilized as an approach to oversee manifestations and improve general prosperity.

During a Reiki session, the expert places their hands either straightforwardly on you or simply above you to achieve mending. The conviction is that the specialist can animate your body's normal mending capacities.

Peruse on to become familiar with the advantages and symptoms of Reiki, and what's in store from a Reiki session.

1. It alleviates agony, uneasiness, and weariness.

As per a survey of randomized trials, Reiki may diminish agony and uneasiness; however, more research is required. It might likewise diminish exhaustion.

A 2015 study found that individuals being treated for malignant growth who got inaccessible Reiki notwithstanding customary therapeutic consideration had lower levels of agony, nervousness, and weariness. These levels were essentially lower than the control gathering, who just got therapeutic consideration. Members had 30-minute sessions of far off Reiki for five days.

In another 2015 investigation, specialists took a gander at the impacts of Reiki on ladies following cesarean conveyance. They found that Reiki fundamentally diminished agony, uneasiness, and the breathing rate in ladies 1-2 days subsequent to having a cesarean conveyance. The requirement for and the number of pain-relieving torment executioners were likewise decreased. Reiki didn't affect circulatory strain or heartbeat rate.

A 2018 study contrasted the utilization of Reiki with physiotherapy for mitigating lower back torment in individuals with herniated plates. The two medications were seen as similarly viable at soothing torment, yet Reiki was savvier and, now and again, brought about quicker treatment.

2. It treats misery.

Reiki medications might be utilized as a feature of a treatment intends to help soothe wretchedness.
In a little 2010 investigation, specialists took a gander at the impacts of Reiki on more seasoned grown-ups encountering agony, despondency, or uneasiness. The members revealed an improvement of their physical indications, state of mind,

and prosperity. They likewise revealed more sentiments of unwinding, expanded interest, and improved degrees of self-care.

3. It improves personal satisfaction.

The positive advantages of Reiki can improve your general prosperity. Analysts in a little 2016 investigation found that Reiki was useful in improving the personal satisfaction for ladies with the disease. Ladies who had Reiki indicated upgrades to their rest designs, fearlessness, and sadness levels. They noticed a feeling of quiet, inward harmony, and unwinding.

4. It helps the state of mind.

Reiki may improve your disposition by diminishing uneasiness and discouragement.
As indicated by results from a recent report, individuals who had Reiki felt a more noteworthy state of mind advantages contrasted with individuals who didn't have Reiki. The investigation members who had six 30-minute sessions over a time of two to about two months demonstrated upgrades in their state of mind.

5. It might improve a few indications and conditions.

Reiki may likewise be utilized to treat:

-Cerebral pain

-Strain

-Sleep deprivation

-Queasiness

The unwinding reaction that occurs with Reiki may profit these indications. In any case, explicit research is expected to decide the adequacy of Reiki for the treatment of these side effects and conditions.

The body is an innately savvy framework. The cells of the body are alive and loaded up with insight. They put forth an admirable attempt to keep the body working in an immaculate request. Infection happens when the cells are worried about such a degree, that they overlook what they are normally intended to do. When you start to make a restorative move, start a discussion with your body or body part. Converse with it as you would converse with a companion.

State, "My Dear Body, I am presently mindful of amazing parts that are not working. We are taking restorative measures to fix them. Much obliged to you for carrying this to my mindfulness through these side effects. You would now be able to return to your common condition of impeccable wellbeing and amicability."

Likewise, demand it to start mending. For this, you can put your hand over the body or body part and state "Mend" in a tone that is instructing yet kind. This will enable the body to realize that you are not kidding about recuperating.

At long last, give up to the procedure. Try not to continue keeping an eye on whether the condition is recuperating. You have done your part. In this way, simply be certain that you will recuperate. Attempting to constrain a recuperating can make more squares en route. Continue doing what you have to do and afterward given up. Trust that when you have the will to mend, you will be bolstered by the Universe and by your own body. When you assume liability, you will likewise be guided if there is something more you have to do to recuperate yourself. Trust that mending will happen in perfect planning.

Essential Oils as Healing Materials

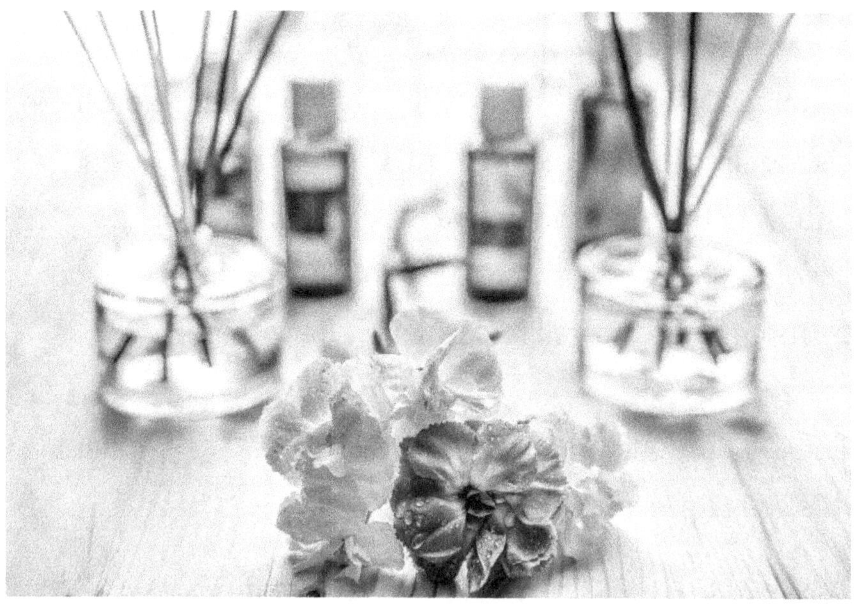

In spite of the fact that fragrance-based treatment is commonly known as an elective treatment, the term integral appears to be all the more fitting as fragrant healing works alongside different modalities including Reiki. The Reiki specialist puts their hands on the customer utilizing light touch and no weight or by putting their hands simply over the customer's body. They work by attracting the vitality of the universe and diverting this positive, recuperating vitality to the customer. The customer may feel this as a warm or shivering sensation in the body.

Utilizing fragrance-based treatment fundamental oils can improve Reiki medicines. Reiki will consistently work for the most noteworthy great, so when utilized with the vitality contained inside basic oils, it will guide the vitality to where it is required and do the greatest. Utilize basic oils in a diffuser in the room where the Reiki treatment will be performed, make a fragrant healing mix to shower around the room while the Reiki treatment is performed.

Here is a portion of the fundamental oils that are frequently utilized in Reiki:

-Citrus fundamental oils (for example, Lemon basic oil, Orange basic oil, Mandarin basic oil, Lime basic oil, and Grapefruit basic oil).

-Lavender fundamental oil

-Sandalwood fundamental oil

-Ylang fundamental oil

Chakra Blends

There are seven chakras or vitality focuses on various pieces of the body. Each chakra is related to a gathering of organs. Cooperating in parity they help keep an individual well. The hand positions utilized in Reiki, spread and treat all major chakras. At the point when Reiki is utilized with fundamental oils identified with the seven noteworthy chakras, together they make a ground-breaking association. Reiki medicines clear the chakras of adverse vitality and blockages, reestablishing the Ki or Chi and helping the individual to recuperate.

Fundamental oils and fragrance-based treatment are progressively being utilized to build the adequacy of other mending modalities; for example, Reiki.

The Relationship of Reiki And Sex

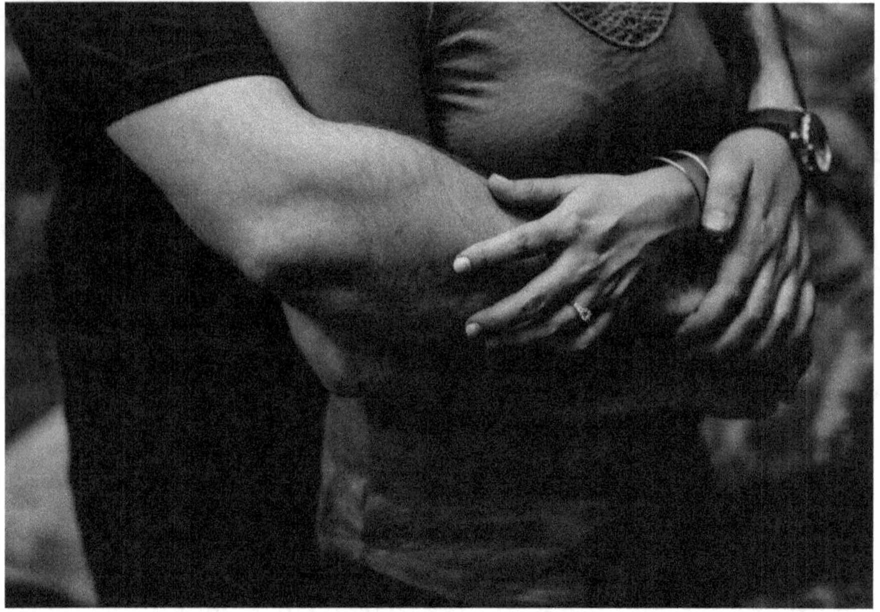

Sex is far beyond that of a definition alone, it is physical, passionate, otherworldly, ceremonial, and much additionally depending who the individual is or their introduction, childhood, and religion.

Reiki, "Widespread Life Force Energy", a recuperating strategy dependent on the rule that the professional can channel vitality into the customer by methods for contact, to actuate the normal mending procedures of the customer's body and reestablish physical and enthusiastic prosperity.

When separating this into the real importance Reiki is two separate words Rei and Ki. Rei, meaning a higher knowledge that aides the creation and working of the universe. Ki, which means the non-physical vitality that enlivens every single living thing.

These interpretations alone are a clarification of how Reiki can conceivably help with recuperating sexual lopsidedness. One thing to recollect is that Reiki can never do any damage.

The sacral chakra decides our sexual cravings and attitude. It is additionally connected with our fun-loving nature and our imaginative natures. Otherworldly exercises related to the sacral chakra are inventiveness, indication, respecting connections, and figuring out how to "let go."

The procedure that enacts Reiki moves the Ki energies through all the chakras. The vitality development starts at the crown chakra and moves to descend through the root chakra and back up once more.

Any chakras that are closed down or in part obstructed be opened during the Reiki session. The second chakra, the body's sexual focus, can't resist the opportunity to be influenced by this. This is particularly valid on the off chance that it has not been working completely previously. On the off chance that an individual has been explicitly subdued or has had his sexual focus closed down, the Reiki session could open up shrouded closeness related issues, sexual inclinations, and feelings.

Everybody can have a functioning sexual coexistence notwithstanding when their sacral chakra is blocked or shut down. Fundamentally, an individual with a shut sexual focus experiences the movement of engaging in sexual relations without having all-out attention to their body. Having intercourse along these lines can be charming, yet it doesn't measure up to having a sexual involvement with the sacral chakra open.

In fact, being completely in your body during sex can be elating, no doubt. You won't almost certainly overlook the inclination once you have encountered it since it is an astounding mix of the physical and the otherworldly.

Reiki Exercise: Beginner

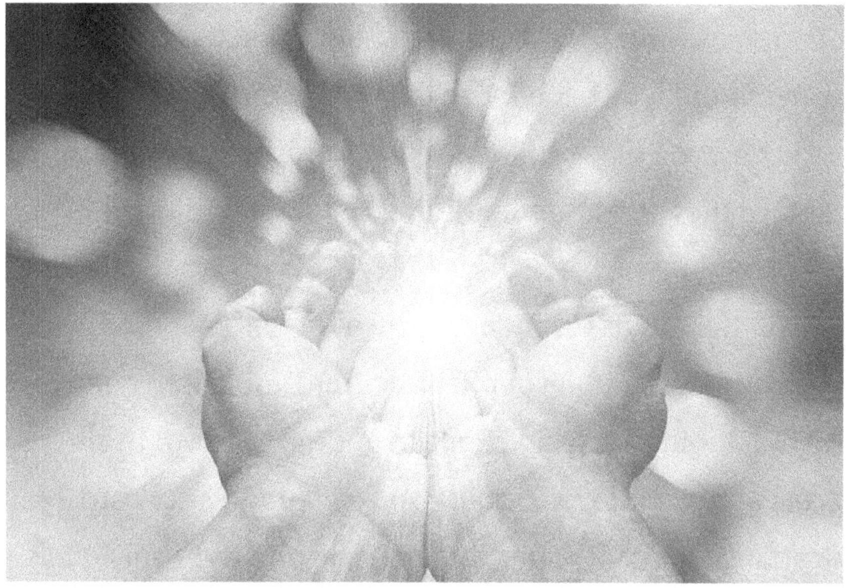

Reiki treatment is an elective recuperating methodology that was created in 1922 by Mikao Usui, a Japanese Buddhist.

It is unwinding and decreases pressure, which all by itself advances recuperating. Be that as it may, there's additional. Professionals use "laying on hands," mantras and gifts to clear the vitality in the body and increment the progression of life power vitality so as to clear the psychological and enthusiastic poisons that meddle with life power vitality and cause issues.

On the off chance that your life power vitality is high and its movement through the body is free and unhindered, life streams easily for you. On the off chance that it is low, or in the event that you experience the ill effects of vitality blockages, you may experience the ill effects of physical and mental issues and undesirable life circumstances.

Reiki for fledglings essentially focuses on self-mending. As you progress through your Reiki venture you might need to find out about overseeing Reiki to another person. This occurs after Reiki level 2 where you will progress toward becoming sensitive to performing Reiki on other individuals. Remember that when you offer Reiki to another person that you effectively clarify the idea of Reiki mending.

This is essentially clarifying what you realized previously. Reiki recuperates sources, not indications. This won't occur immediately however may take numerous Reiki sessions to completely address the foundation of the issue.

Furthermore, it is imperative to make a patient completely mindful of the 'purging period'. This is fundamentally the same as what you yourself experienced after attunement in

Reiki for tenderfoots level 1, or even after level 2. Manifestations can become more grounded as the patient's body and mind participate with oneself recuperating mechanics of Reiki. Clarify that an individual can experience changes over their life and that occasionally these might be concentrated. They may notice signs in their lives that reveal to them what ways or bearings they ought to take, what isn't helping their lives in any case and would be in an ideal situation halted, who contributes and who detracts from their lives. It is imperative to clarify these in detail generally a patient may get frightened and stop Reiki treatment.

Likewise, attempt to decide whether an individual truly wishes to be mended. A few people simply would prefer not to show signs of improvement for reasons unknown. Have a long discourse with the patient and figure out what their expectations are. In the event that an individual doesn't wish to be recuperated, at that point, Reiki won't affect them.

This is an outline of what you'll have to comprehend in Reiki for apprentices. To advance on your adventure don't hesitate to peruse the various articles on this site to build your comprehension and see the numerous advantages Reiki can bring into a people life.

Reiki Exercise: Intermediate

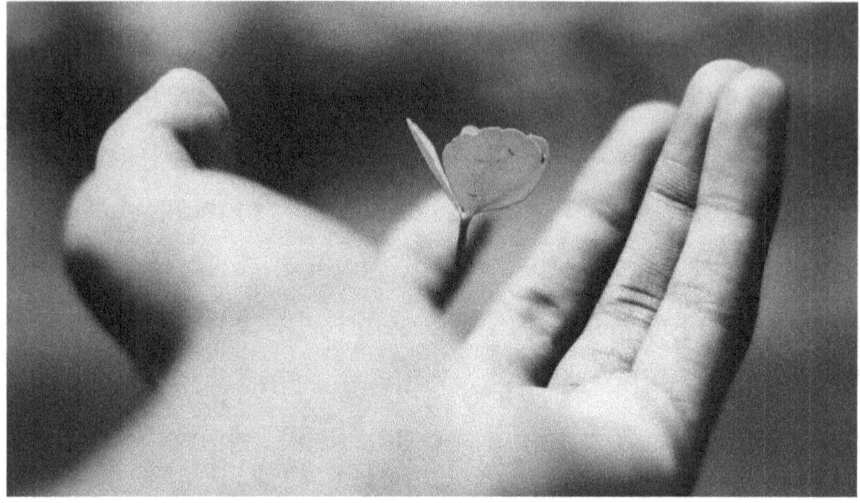

The quality and estimation of the Reiki practice you perform can be improved by observing some essential standards. There are various things you can in like manner do that will construct the nature of our Reiki. Remember, Reiki begins from an unlimited stock and contains the venerating learning of the most critical significant power. There is no limitation to the bit of leeway and worth that is doable for you to get from Reiki. As you endeavor the strategies in this book, plan that they will work for you and know in your heart this is right and you will get the improved results you search for.

The idea of the imperativeness in the room you do your Reiki drugs in is critical at whatever point improved results are what you search for. Guarantee the room isn't unnecessarily hot or too much cool. Guarantee there is characteristic air from an open window or that the room isn't stuffy. A clean and tidy room is also helpful as negative perceptive essentialness will, as a rule, assemble around disturbance and wreckage Smudge the stay with sage when treatment releases any negative energies left by past clients and to go about it as a blessing. As you smear, get the antecedents and the climbed managers and Reiki associates mentioning that they support you and your client and to help you with your recovering treatment. Spot pictures of Dr. Usui, Dr. Hayashi, and Mrs. Takata around the room and solicitation that they are accessible. The use of incense, essential oils or new blossoms will in like manner act to raise the vibration. Moderating music during the treatment will empower the client to move into a continuously responsive point of view.

Before the client comes, sit in an intelligent state with your hands on your legs doing Reiki on yourself. By then after several minutes, use your order hand to enthusiastically draw the Reiki Power picture in light on every divider, and on the rooftop and floor.

As you do this state "I support this existence with light" on various occasions for each spot. By then draw the power picture in the point of convergence of the room and send Reiki into the space to fill the existence with recovering essentialness. You can similarly send evacuated Reiki to your client while they are in transit to the session so they will be free and in an open state when they appear.

Preceding starting the treatment, place the power and expert pictures on your palm chakras. This will even more absolutely open the palm chakras and invigorate them. By then draw a gigantic power picture down the front of your body to guarantee and connect with you and draw tinier power pictures on each chakra. Placing the pictures into the clients crown chakra, and seeing them go into the client's heart is moreover significant before starting as it raises the vibration of the treatment and makes the essentialness of the pictures progressively open.

It is a captivating component of Reiki that when giving a treatment, Reiki will continue spilling paying little regard to what you do with your mind.

You can talk with others about any subject - including unimportant issues, or snitch or even visit on the phone and

Reiki will continue to stream and the client will get some bit of leeway. Nevertheless, this sort of lead doesn't convey the best results with Reiki. It must be recalled that giving Reiki is a significant experience and is even more appropriately given with reverence. By thinking about the movement of Reiki as it experiences you, rather than talking, you won't simply encounter the essentialness even more clearly, yet will similarly assemble its stream. As you think about the Reiki essentialness, your mind joins with it and causes your imperativeness field to resound in increasingly unmistakable concurrence with the movement of Reiki, along these lines empowering it to stream even more transparently. As you do this, you may feel streams of essentialness coursing through various bits of your body including your spine, chakras, arms, and hands. You may moreover feel the warmth, quieting sensations, vibrations, throbs or surges of essentialness experiencing you. By using your internal eye, you may similarly have the choice to see the Reiki imperativeness. This may appear as unobtrusive particles of white or splendid light or various shades of imperativeness coursing through you.

As you might suspect and unite with these sensations, your mind will be motivated, twisting up progressively optimistic.

Opinions of enjoyment, concordance, and significant love will be experienced. Radiantly positive dreams and dreams of higher significant planes can similarly be experienced. By going interior and looking upward through your crown chakra, it is even possible to supernaturally go up to the wellspring of Reiki and unite with it. All of these experiences are really charming and can be significantly repairing for the expert while they increase the favorable position to the client. As you think about Reiki thusly, you will moreover be opening the pathways through which Reiki can stream, as such growing the nature of Reiki you are redirecting to your client. This is a really beguiling way to deal with improve the idea of the Reiki you give.

Adding supplication to your Reiki prescriptions is furthermore a fruitful strategy that will grow its quality. While you are giving a treatment, you can ask undeniably or to yourself.
Approach the climbed Reiki specialists, or on Jesus, St. Germain, Buddha, Krishna, Babaji, or other rose specialists, favored delegates, or soul oversees, or ask direct to the unending God/Goddess or to the Reiki essentialness itself. As you supplicate, ask that your Reiki be braced and demand that it supports you and your client. Solicitation supports and

guides your Reiki practice. This is to guide you in extending its quality and the favorable position it gives you and those you treat. Recognize the path that there is no limitation to the value and recovering influence that is open to you and ask that you be regarded with an abundance of patching, appreciating significant essentialness so you will be of increasingly imperative help to other individuals. Solidify your petitions with the above methodology of combining with the essentialness and feeling it as it travels through you. By begging as you do Reiki, your supplications will be even more predominant since when doing Reiki, you are even more clearly connected with the more dominant which is the wellspring of all tended to appeal.

Drawing on an uncommon patching aide or aides that will work with you will in like manner improve your prescriptions. While Reiki comes authentically from God, there are supernatural assistants who are capable of healing.

They can add their Reiki energies to yours and moreover channel Reiki clearly to the client.
Many have uncovered that they felt additional hands on them and the closeness of someone else in the room during a Reiki treatment. Needing to help and supplicating that a

recovering assistant or glorious specialist will come to empower you can accomplish this. In like manner, using the "Meet Your Reiki Guides" copied in the flyer can make this affiliation.

Reiki Exercise: Advance

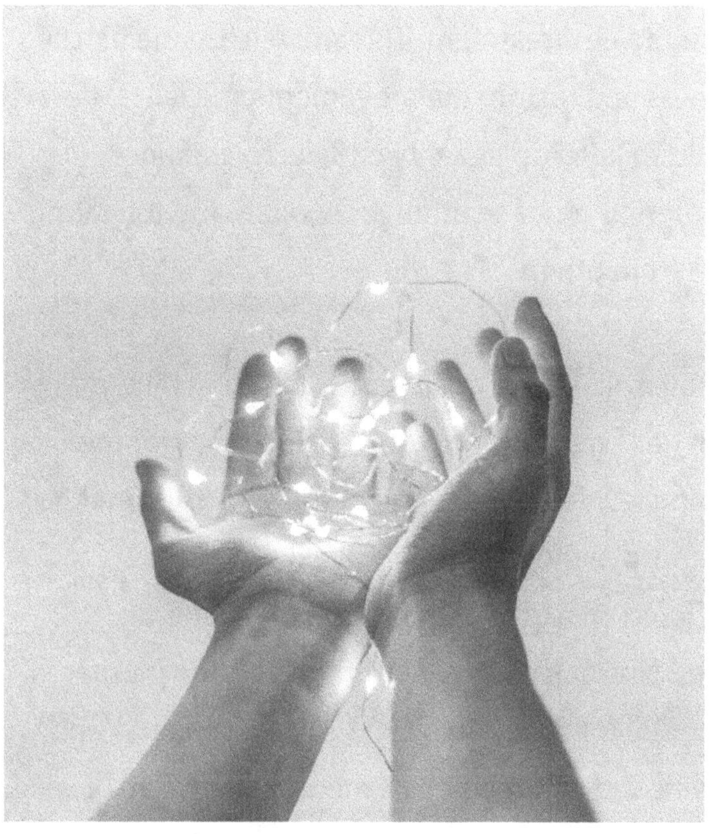

Some Reiki experts report that their Reiki seems to have lost a part of its ability and they wonder why this happens and what should be conceivable to get it back. When doing Reiki, the master moreover gets a treatment. Right when this happens, to a great extent negative essentialness is loose and begins to go through the masters' structure on out.

This essentialness can once in a while slow down out by chance so ones Reiki will by and large work on the authority more than gushing to other individuals. What is required is for the master to get treatment. This will release the blocked imperativeness and restore the movement of Reiki. Review that, we need to keep up equality of Reiki by treating ourselves, offering drugs to other individuals and tolerating medications from others.

Your Reiki can in like manner increase when you take your next level of Reiki getting ready. The attunement for the accompanying level and the usage of the symbol(s) that go with it can improve the idea of your Reiki drugs. This is routinely offered an explanation to occur by general understudies. One authority reported that his life partner was in perpetual torment, which was simply generally and fleetingly removed with his Reiki II meds. In the wake of taking the Master setting one up, treatment using the Master picture completely released the torment and it didn't return. Your Reiki can in like manner improve by tolerating additional attunements for a comparable level you are starting at now have.

In spite of the way that you need only a solitary attunement to have Reiki for marvelous advantages, extra attunements for a comparative level you have will further refine and strengthen your Reiki. Various Masters will give extra attunements in vain or for a low cost. A portion of the time new Masters need people to practice on, don't hesitate to volunteer.

A social affair of Masters can practice attunements on each other and strengthen their Reiki at the same time. Have each Master give the Master attunement to each person in the social affair. If you have five Masters, by then, each will get four Master attunements and give four. This can be incredibly stunning.

Chi Gong and Tai Chi are techniques for structuring up your Chi and opening the pathways that Chi or Ki courses through. The pathways that are opened in these exercises are comparable ones that Reiki travels through. On the ordinary, a large number of individuals who have penetrated this kind of moving consideration have more grounded Reiki than the people who have not.

Find an educator you feel incredible with and take up the typical daily practice concerning Chi Gong or Tai Chi and not solely will it be sound for you; be that as it may, your Reiki will in like manner improve.

It is possible to use self-enchanting and examination similarly as requests to improve your Reiki. Basically, enter self-hypnotizing or thought and prescribe to yourself that your Reiki is getting more grounded and more grounded and more grounded and it will. You can in like manner do this while giving a treatment.

Playing the "Discussing Reiki Masters" tape while giving a treatment can in like manner improve the estimation of your Reiki. The tape was made by 18 Reiki Masters who discussed the names of all of the four Reiki pictures into a recipient while arranging that all who hear the sound will be retouched. Most who play the tape while giving a treatment see an improvement in the idea of their Reiki.

Placing blessed pictures in your Reiki room when you are doing Reiki can in like manner construct the estimation of your prescriptions.
This consolidates pictures of Jesus, Buddha, Krishna or some other significant teacher or mind boggling being. The Beaming Reiki Masters picture in the back of "Reiki, The Healing Touch" will in like manner raise the vibration of your meds similarly as the Antakarana that is given in the Master getting ready. You can put these cards under your Reiki table

or on the mass of your retouching room.

Reiki attunements open and extend the Ki-holding limit or the Hara Line and clear vitality blockages. They open a channel for the Reiki vitality to spill out of professional to customer. The more a professional uses Reiki the clearer and more grounded the stream progresses toward becoming. The attunement procedure is the thing that makes Reiki stand separated from different sorts of recuperating frameworks. Albeit other mending expressions may utilize hand positions on the customer, just Reiki has the magnificent advantage of the attunement procedure.

Reiki specialists will regularly make a loosening up air for their Reiki sessions, setting the state of mind with the utilization of diminished lights, thoughtful music, or percolating drinking fountains.
A few professionals like to be in a spot that is totally quiet, without the interruption of music of any sort, to lead their Reiki sessions in. Consequently, you can't learn Reiki through finding out about it; it must be experienced. Be that as it may, the business sectors are flooding with an ever-increasing number of enlightening books expounded on Reiki. Reiki can turn into a lifestyle if that is what you think

about it.

These are a few procedures for improving the nature of your Reiki. Endeavor them. In like manner, remember that Reiki has its very own awareness and by basically proposing to find ways to deal with improve the value you pass on to others with your meds, and by being accessible to its heading, the Reiki imperativeness will oversee you to additional ways. Reiki begins from an interminable stock. There is no confinement to the retouching power that is open to you. Focus on reverence and sympathy. Trust in your internal direction and make a move on it. You won't be baffled.

Conclusion

Thank for making it through to the end of " Reiki Healing For Beginners: Heal yourself and the others, increase your energy, improve your health, reduce stress and unlock the secret about physical, mental, emotional and spiritual therapy." , we should trust it was enlightening and ready to give all of you of the instruments you have to accomplish your objectives whatever it is that they might be. Because you've completed this book doesn't mean there is nothing left to learn on the theme, extending your points of view is the best way to discover the authority you look for.

The subsequent stage is to quit perusing and to get beginning doing whatever it is that you have to do so as to guarantee that those you care about will be appropriately dealt with should the need emerge. On the off chance that you find that despite everything, you need assistance beginning you will probably have better outcomes by making a timetable that you plan to pursue including exacting cutoff times for different pieces of the errands just as the general consummation of your arrangements.

Studies demonstrate that mind-boggling undertakings that are separated into individual pieces, including singular cutoff times, have a lot more prominent shot of being finished when contrasted with something that has a general need of being finished yet no ongoing table for doing as such. Regardless of whether it appears to be senseless, feel free to set your own cutoff times for consummation, complete with pointers of progress and disappointment. After you have effectively finished the majority of your required arrangements you will be happy you did.

When you have completed your underlying arrangements for Reiki Self-Treatment, comprehend that they are only that, the lone piece of a bigger arrangement of readiness. Your best shots for general achievement will be stopped by setting aside the effort to learn whatever number fundamental aptitudes as could be allowed, which will be incorporated into our different books concerning the body's Chakra System. Just by utilizing your readied status as a springboard to the more noteworthy arrangement, will you have the option to really rest adequately realizing that you are set up for everything without exception that life chooses to toss at you?

At last, in the event that you discovered this book helpful in any case, a survey on Amazon is constantly valued!

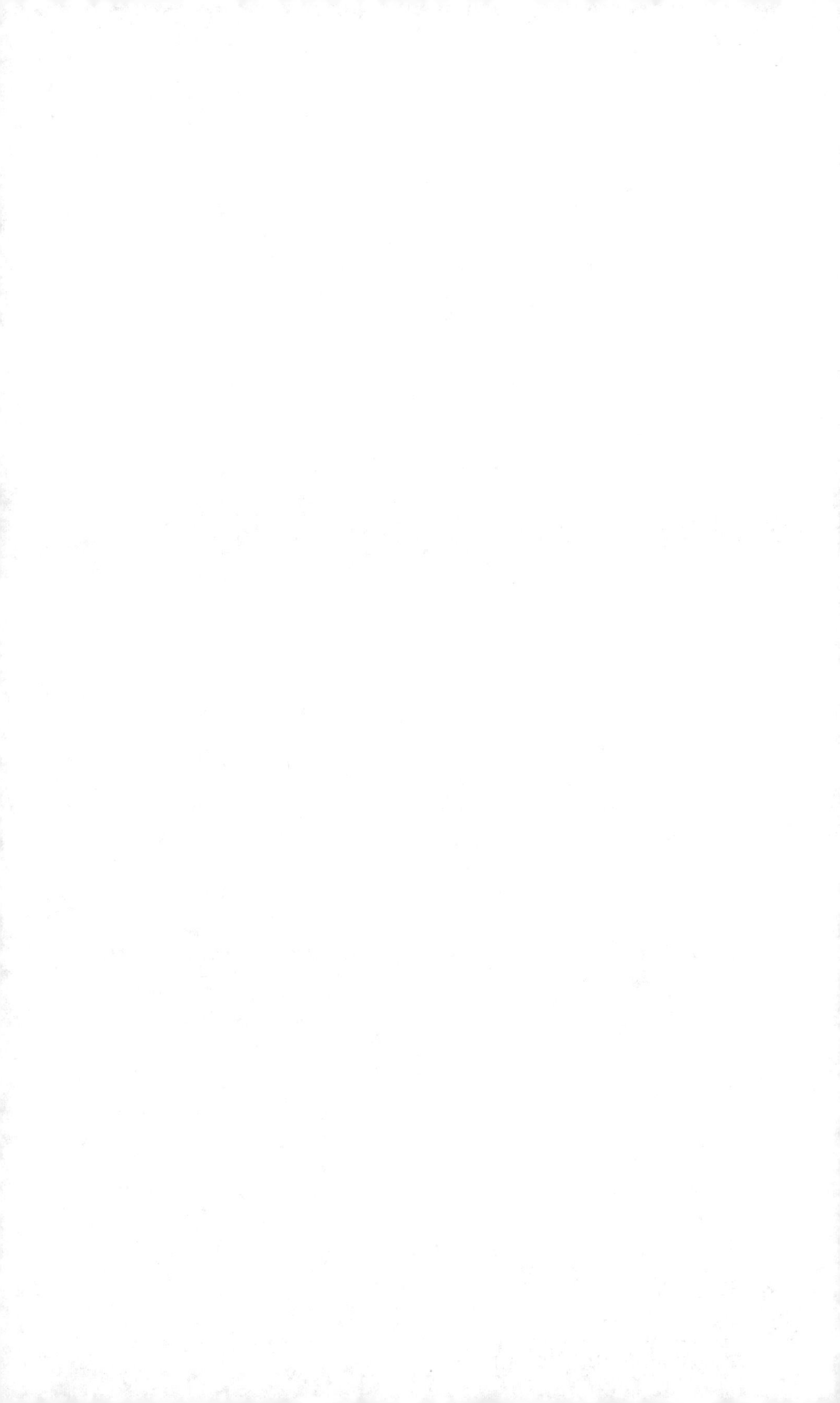